Innovative Implantation Technique

Marie-José Tassignon
Sorcha Ní Dhubhghaill • Luc Van Os
Editors

Innovative Implantation Technique

Bag-in-the-Lens Cataract Surgery

Springer

Editors
Marie-José Tassignon
Department of Ophthalmology
Antwerp University, University Hospital
Edegem
Belgium

Sorcha Ní Dhubhghaill
Department of Ophthalmology
Antwerp University, University Hospital
Edegem
Belgium

Luc Van Os
Department of Ophthalmology
Antwerp University, University Hospital
Edegem
Belgium

ISBN 978-3-030-03085-8 ISBN 978-3-030-03086-5 (eBook)
https://doi.org/10.1007/978-3-030-03086-5

Library of Congress Control Number: 2018968144

This Springer imprint is published by the registered company Springer Nature Switzerland AG
The registered company address is: Gewerbestrasse 11, 6330 Cham, Switzerland

Contents

Part I

Why Use the BIL?

The History of the Bag-in-the-Lens Implant

1

Marie-José Tassignon

1.1 Introduction

Back in 1999, I had the honor of meeting Sir Harold Ridley in Stockholm on the occasion of the European Society of Ophthalmology (SOE) meeting. He and his wife Elisabeth were guests of honor at the European Society meeting. I hoped to take advantage of this opportunity to discuss the concept of the bag-in-the-lens. Given that he was about 90 years of age, I realized that this was a "mission impossible" and felt satisfied with a picture in his company (Fig. 1.1). I wanted to explain some thoughts that I had on modifying, very slightly, his original design, which was round with a small edge surrounding the lens optic (Fig. 1.2). In the original drawings and publications [1–2], the Ridley lens was clearly intended to be positioned within the capsular bag and to fill this bag as much as possible. However, I still had the question of why such funny edges were placed at the periphery of the lens optic. My idea was to make that edge longer and to extend it out from both the anterior and posterior surfaces of the lens optic. This would create a groove between the flanges that could accommodate both the anterior and posterior capsules.

David Apple, professor of ophthalmology and pathology at Moran Eye Center, Salt Lake City, Utah, USA, dedicated a lot of his time to writing a bibliography of Harold Ridley [3]. He traveled to England many times to meet Sir Harold Ridley, not just as a colleague but as a personal friend. He was eager to hear the master describe his account of the discovery of the intraocular lens that would revolutionize cataract surgery worldwide in person.

In Chap. 11 of David Apple's book [3], Harold Ridley reported secondary cataract and lens "decentration" as "modern" cataract surgery's most common

M.-J. Tassignon (✉)
Department of Ophthalmology, Antwerp University, University Hospital, Edegem, Belgium
e-mail: marie-jose.tassignon@uza.be

M.-J. Tassignon et al. (eds.), *Innovative Implantation Technique*,
https://doi.org/10.1007/978-3-030-03086-5_1

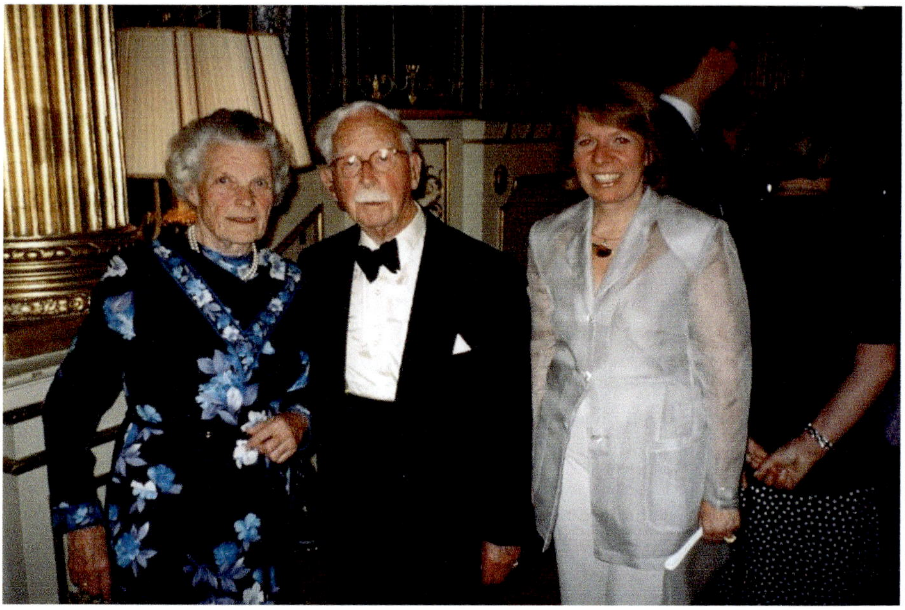

Fig. 1.1 With Harold Ridley and his wife Elisabeth at SOE in Stockholm 1999

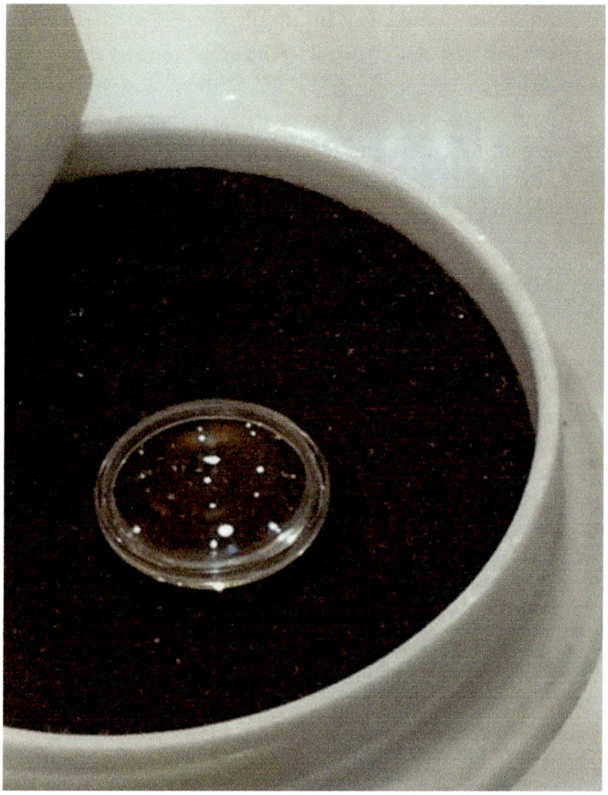

Fig. 1.2 Harold Ridley's first IOL design, manufactured by Rayner[R], UK

postoperative surgical complications. The quest to solve these problems with the bag-in-the-lens began there.

Charles Kelman was a dear friend and mentor to me. He supported me on my quest to write the patent on the bag-in-the-lens and invited me, every year, to be a speaker at the "French Phaco courses," organized in New York. The aim of these French Phaco courses was to disseminate his message about the superiority of the phaco technique to the international community of French-speaking ophthalmologists in the USA. Charles Kelman spoke fluent French, since he spent many years in a French-speaking canton in Switzerland. He put me in contact with his attorney, who helped me in the administrative follow-up of the BIL patent which was issued in February 2000 [4]. It was remarkable to remember, from Charles Kelman's oral presentations, that although the phaco technique improved the surgical outcome dramatically, the most frequent complications remained. These included (Fig. 1.3):

1. Opacification of the lens capsular bag, which was ultimately referred to as posterior capsule opacification or PCO
2. Loss of accommodation (interest in restoring accommodation became reality starting from the mid-1990s on)

More than 40 years after the introduction of the first intraocular lens implantation and the advent of the phaco technique, PCO was still the most common complication after cataract surgery until Daniele Aron-Rosa [5] and Franz Fankhauser [6] came up with the disruptive Q-switched Nd-YAG laser, to mechanically open the opacified capsular bag. I knew Daniele Aron-Rosa as an excellent scientist with a warm personality. She was also very interested in art, and one of her hobbies was

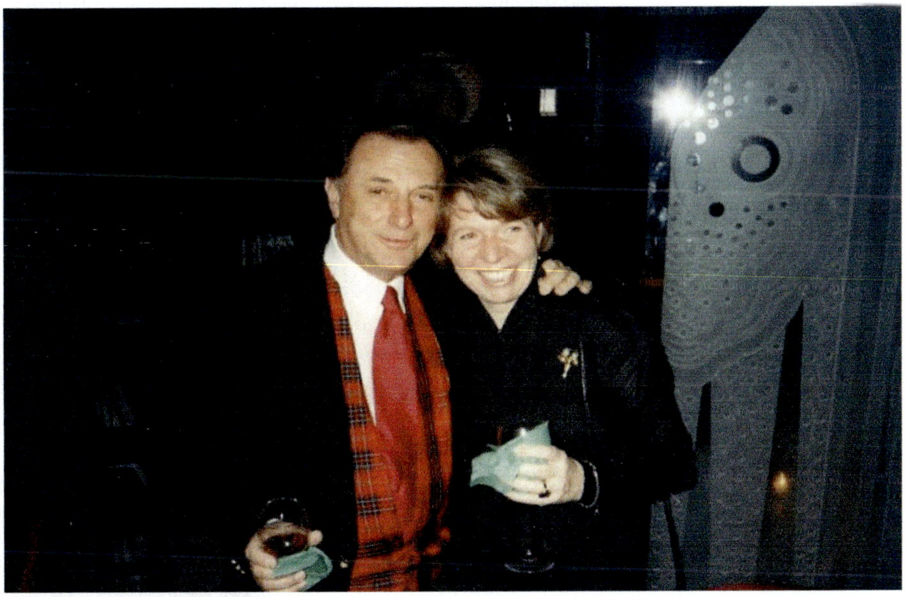

Fig. 1.3 With Charles Kelman in New York, 1998

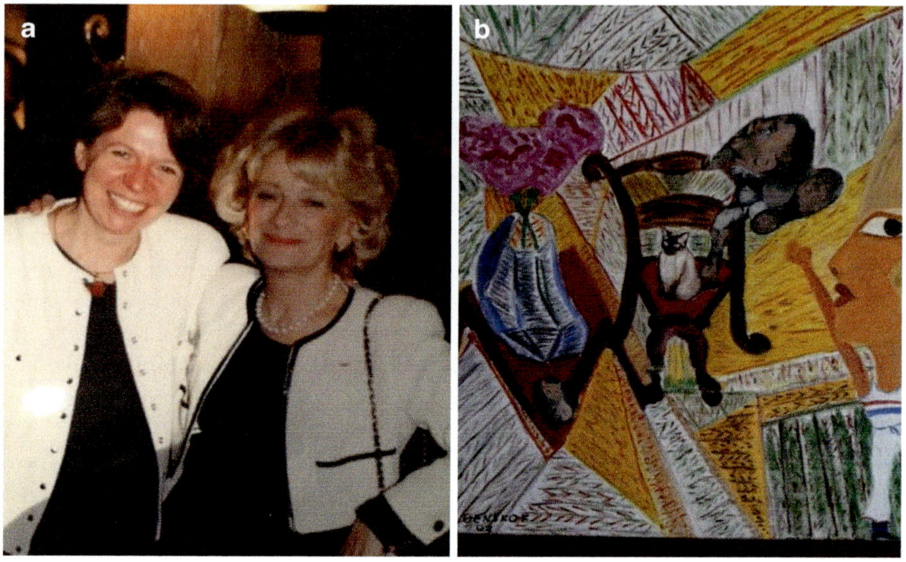

Fig. 1.4 (**a**) With Daniele Aron-Rosa in 2003 and (**b**) one of her paintings signed Genskof of that same period

painting. Her artist's name is Genskof, and I was fortunate to receive one of her paintings through a common friend, Dr. René Trau, in 2003 (Fig. 1.4). Franz Fankhauser's Q-switched Nd-YAG laser machine presented more treatment options than that of Aron-Rosa, and although I was not directly connected to him, he inspired me to use the laser to treat vitreal problems like premacular hemorrhages and floaters. The latter is now drawing a great deal of attention in ophthalmological practice, and while I will not elaborate on that topic here, I am of the opinion that floaters are very important in cataract surgery, particularly when using complex optics such as multifocal IOLs. The quality of the image, as perceived by the patient, will be influenced negatively by the presence of floaters.

Even though Nd-YAG laser capsulotomy was a real leap forward in modern cataract surgery, the effect of the foreign body reaction of the intraocular lens biomaterial on the capsular bag had not yet been solved. Our department showed that while performing a YAG laser could clear the visual axis, a significant amount of higher-order aberrations remained which indicated that Nd-YAG treatment did not provide as good an image, as there had been no PCO at all. We demonstrated that the incidence of ocular aberrations decreased but remained quite high compared to the immediate postoperative measurements [7]. Patient's quality of the image is, therefore, still suboptimal following Nd-YAG laser capsulotomy, even if the visual axis is optimally transparent to light. It became clear to me that while visual acuity can be excellent, patients may still suffer from a poor but sufficient "quality of vision." This new concept plays an important role when trying to understand why patients are unhappy after an uneventful cataract surgery and an implantation of an intraocular lens with complex optics.

1.2 BIL Concept

The BIL intraocular lens is "suspended" by the lens capsule, while the intraocular lens is inserted into the capsule bag (Fig. 1.5a) in the lens-in-the-bag method. At the core of the bag-in-the-lens principle is the sequestration of the lens epithelial cells of the inner plane of the anterior lens capsule and of the equatorial area of the crystalline lens into the sealed lens capsule (Fig. 1.5b, (a and b)). The area of contact of

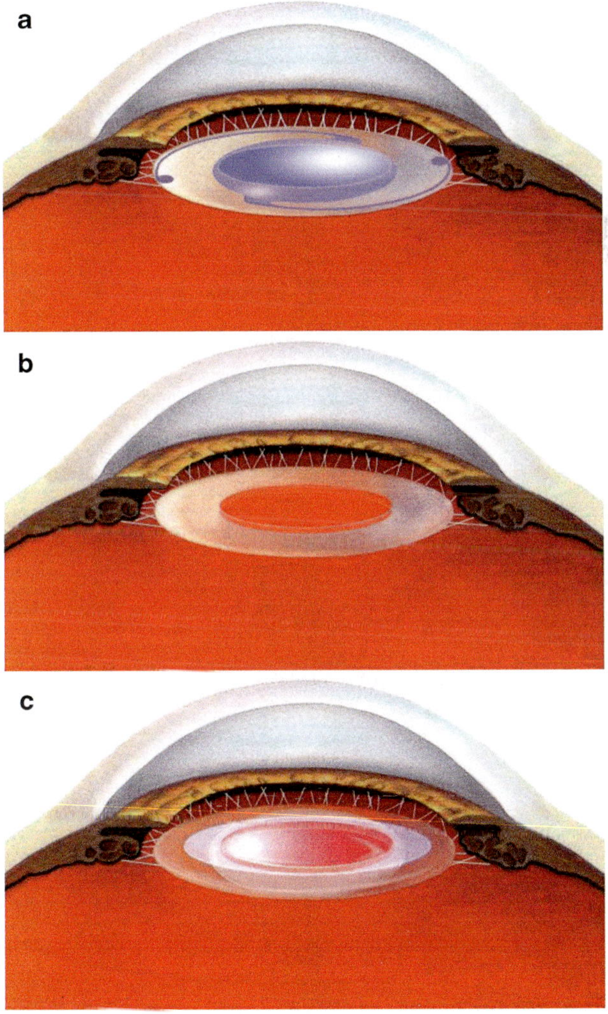

Fig. 1.5 Differences in concept in (**a**) the lens-in-the-bag in which the intraocular lens is inserted into the capsule bag and (**b**) the bag-in-the-lens implantation techniques where an anterior and posterior capsulorhexis is performed of similar size (a) in order to insert both together into the lens groove surrounding the lens optic (b). (Drawings made by R. Leysen)

the capsule bag (and accompanying lens epithelial cells) with the biomaterial of the intraocular lens is very large in the traditional lens-in-bag approach, while the contact of the biomaterial with the lens capsule is reduced to the lens groove with the bag-in-the-lens method. This major difference explains why the lens epithelial cells undergo very little metaplasia into myofibroblasts in the bag-in-the-lens implantation technique.

George Duncan from Norwich University (UK) and later on Michael Wormstone (Norwich, UK) spent a lot of their careers in exploring the mechanism behind

US006027531A

United States Patent [19]
Tassignon

[11] **Patent Number:** **6,027,531**
[45] **Date of Patent:** **Feb. 22, 2000**

[54] **INTRAOCULAR LENS AND METHOD FOR PREVENTING SECONDARY OPACIFICATION**

[76] Inventor: **Marie-José B. R. Tassignon**, Wapenhaghestraat 10 IN 2600, Berchem-Antwerp, Belgium

[21] Appl. No.: **08/950,290**

[22] Filed: **Oct. 14, 1997**

[51] **Int. Cl.**[7] **A61F 2/16**
[52] **U.S. Cl.** **623/6**; 623/4; 128/898
[58] **Field of Search** 623/6, 4; 128/898

[56] **References Cited**

U.S. PATENT DOCUMENTS

4,485,499	12/1984	Castleman .
4,547,915	10/1985	Castleman .
4,808,181	2/1989	Kelman .
5,002,571	3/1991	O'Donnell, Jr. et al. .
5,366,501	11/1994	Langerman .
5,370,687	12/1994	Poler .
5,405,385	4/1995	Heimke et al. .
5,445,636	8/1995	Bretton .
5,549,670	8/1996	Young et al. .
5,576,345	11/1996	Mangnasson .
5,593,438	1/1997	Akhavi et al. .
5,697,973	12/1997	Peyman et al. 623/6

Primary Examiner—David H. Willse
Assistant Examiner—Dinh X. Nguyen
Attorney, Agent, or Firm—Darby & Darby

[57] **ABSTRACT**

An intraocular lens for use in extracapsular cataract extraction has a haptic pat that surrounds the optical pat of the lens and further contains a groove of such shape to accommodate the anterior and posterior capsules of the lens bag after anterior capsulorhexis, extracapsular cataract extraction and posterior capsulorhexis. The lens is preferably inserted in a calibrated, circular and continuous combined anterior and posterior capsulorhexis, slightly smaller than the inner circumference of the groove as to induce a stretching of the rims of the capsular openings. This new approach is believed to prevent the appearance of secondary opacification of the capsules, allows a very stable fixation of the intraocular lens and ensures a tight separation between the anterior and posterior segment of the eye. This new principle of insertion is called the bag-in-the-lens technique, in contrast with the classical lens in-the-bag technique.

8 Claims, 2 Drawing Sheets

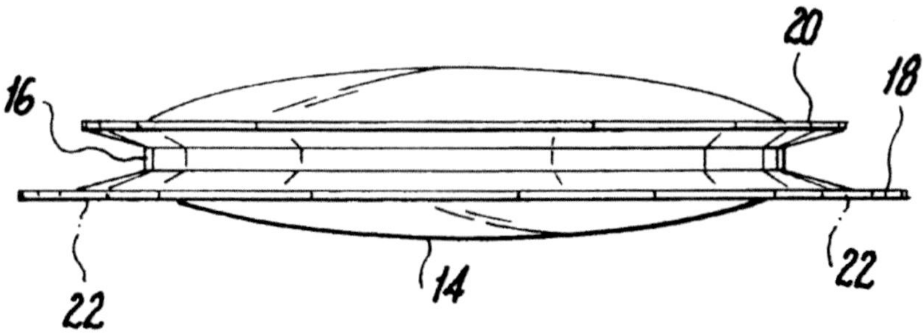

Fig. 1.6 Technical drawing made by Rudi Leysen for the US patent application of the bag-in-the lens

PCO [8]. Based on their studies, it became clear to me that the lens epithelial cells are very potent cells. The message was to keep them far away from cytokines or any other proteins that could trigger their transformation into myofibroblasts, causing fibrotic reaction and contraction of the capsular bag, while the lens epithelial cells keep the capsular bag flexible and transparent under normal physiological circumstances.

The idea of the bag-in-the-lens design came to me as I was listening to George Duncan's lecture in Amsterdam in 1997. I sketched out a drawing on a napkin, and I tried to explain the principle to Jan Worst and Albert Galant during a coffee break. Unfortunately, neither of them paid much attention to the concept. As I was traveling home by train, I sketched out the draft in greater detail, and the next day, I gave it to my very dear and close friend and co-worker Rudi Leysen (medical photographer at the department of the Antwerp University Hospital). He came up with the first technical drawing which I used for the US patent application (Fig. 1.6).

1.3 The Space of Berger

I knew about the different compartments of the vitreous body [9] based on the work of Jan Worst from Groningen, the Netherlands (Fig. 1.7), and more specifically of the presence of the space of Berger [10]. The space of Berger was first described by

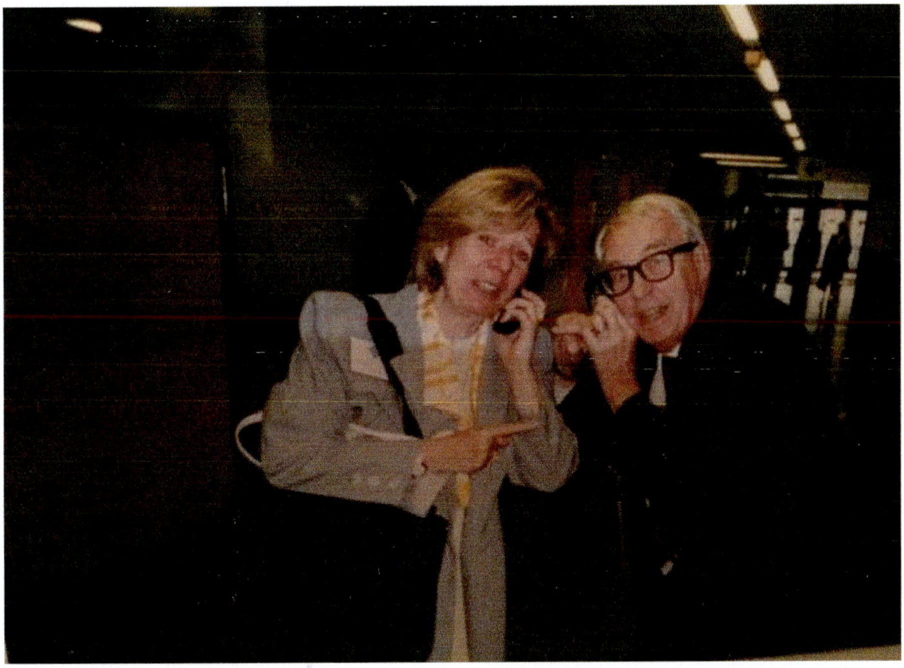

Fig. 1.7 With Prof. Jan Worst at ESCRS meeting in Vienna in 1999

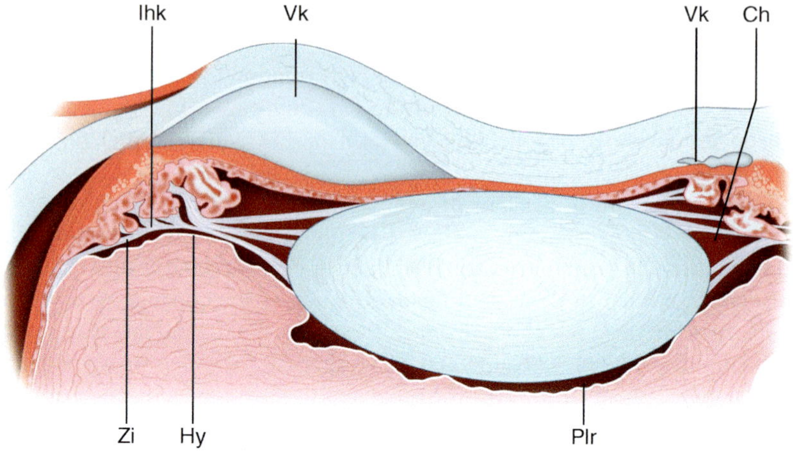

Fig. 1.8 Drawing by Emil Berger of the space defined between the posterior capsule and the anterior hyaloid, later on referred to as the space of Berger. (p 29–30 of Ref. [8])

the ophthalmologist Emil Berger from Graz, Austria. In his thesis, he made a drawing of this area located behind the crystalline lens and beautifully showed how the crystalline lens is completely immersed in water (Fig. 1.8). This space is extremely important to the bag-in-the-lens concept since it accommodates the posterior haptic flange of the lens. The total diameter of the posterior bag-in-the-lens flange haptic is, therefore, no larger than 7.5 mm since the space of Berger in adults is typically about 8–9 mm wide.

We will elaborate more on the importance of this space later in this book as well as on the new discoveries we have been able to make based on our clinical observations while performing a primary posterior continuous circular capsulorhexis routinely in adults and in children [11].

1.4 Conclusion

This book covers 26 years of research, which coincides with my 26-year chairmanship of the department of ophthalmology of the Antwerp University and of the Antwerp University Hospital in Belgium. Prior to this research, I was very active in discovering the effect of lasers on the retina and the vitreous, which was the topic of my PhD thesis defended in Leiden University in 1990. My best man at my PhD defense was Dr. Nikolaas Stempels, a young staff member at the University of Brussels at which I was senior staff at that time. I must thank him for his very supportive role and the many evenings we spent together in brainstorming about the most challenging ideas in the field of ophthalmology.

I have been lucky enough to have met some giants in ophthalmology. They have helped me in finding the answers I was looking for.

At Antwerp University, I was blessed to be surrounded by staff who never faltered in their belief in this novel idea of the bag-in-the-lens. They were instrumental in co-conducting the laboratory and clinical research which generated the reputation of scientific excellence that accompanied this endeavor throughout. I will always be extremely thankful to Veva De Groot, Ilse De Veuster, Jan Van Looveren, Stefan Kiekens, Luc Van Os, and Sorcha Ní Dhubhghaill.

References

1. Ridley NHL. Lenses after cataract extraction. Lancet. 1952;259:118–29.
2. Ridley NHL. Intraocular acrylic lenses -a recent development in the surgery of cataract. Br J Ophthalmol. 1952;36:113–22.
3. Apple DJ. Sir Harold Ridley and his fight for sight. Thorofare: Slack; 2006.
4. MJBR Tassignon, Intraocular lens and method for preventing secondary opacification, US Patent 6,027,531, Feb. 22, 2000.
5. Aron-Rosa D, Aron JJ, Griesemann M, Thyzel R. Use of the neodymium-YAG laser to open the posterior capsule after lens implant surgery: a preliminary report. J Am Intraocul Implant Soc. 1980;6(4):352–4.
6. Fankhauser F, Roussel P, Steffen J. Clinical studies on the efficiency of high power laser radiation upon some structures of the anterior segment of the eye. First experiences of the treatment of some pathological conditions of the anterior segment of the human eye by means of a Qswitched. Int Ophthalmol. 1981;3(3):129–39.
7. Rozema J, Tassignon MJ. Influence of Nd:YAG laser on higher order aberrations after hydrophobic/hydrophilic IOL implantation. J Cataract Refract Surg. 2009;35:1906–10.
8. Wormstone IM. Posterior capsule opacification: a cell biological perspective. Exp Eye Res. 2002;74(3):337–47.
9. Worst JGF, Los LI. Cisternal anatomy of the vitreous. Amsterdam/New York: Kugler Publications; 1995.
10. Berger E. Beitraege zur Anatomie des Auges in normalem und pathologischem Zustande. 1st ed. Wiesbaden: JF Bergmann; 1887.
11. Tassignon MJ, Ni Dhubhghaill S. Real time optical coherence tomography imaging confirms older concepts about the Berger space. Ophthalmic Res. 2016;56:222–6.

Advantages of the Bag-in-the-Lens Implant

2

Sorcha Ní Dhubhghaill

2.1 Introduction

The bag-in-the-lens (BIL) implant was originally designed with the goal of preventing posterior capsular opacification (PCO) in the paediatric population for which the management of secondary cataract can be challenging [1]. Once the concept was proven in paediatric cases [2], the technique was also validated in adults in accordance with the European ISO normative standards [3]. The surgery includes a number of extra steps that are not required in standard cataract surgery, such as a calibrated anterior capsulorhexis and a posterior capsulorhexis.

These additional steps also confer an extra learning curve and as such can incur risks. We have to look this technique's advantages when we consider whether these extra steps and learning curve are worth the additional effort. The aim of this chapter is to provide an overview of the features of the BIL that convinced us to undertake the learning curve and led us to adopt it as our lens of choice for cataract surgery (Fig. 2.1).

S. Ní Dhubhghaill (✉)
Department of Ophthalmology, Antwerp University, University Hospital, Edegem, Belgium

M.-J. Tassignon et al. (eds.), *Innovative Implantation Technique*,
https://doi.org/10.1007/978-3-030-03086-5_2

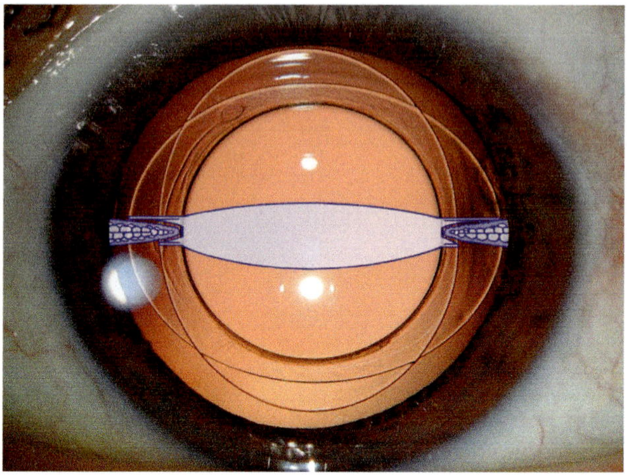

Fig. 2.1 The BIL implant in situ with a schematic overlay of the lens in profile

2.2 Indications for a BIL

The implantation of a BIL is possible in most cases of cataract surgery as an alternative to the standard in the bag approach. We use this lens for all standard cataract cases. There are cases for which additional care must be taken, however. Patients with a small iris, history of trauma or zonular weakness all require extra care.

2.3 Advantages of the BIL

The first main advantage of the lens is the prevention of PCO. When correctly implanted, the lens design mechanically prevents the normal migration of lens epithelial cells over the posterior surface of the intraocular lens [4]. When I present this technique publicly, I say that I have no financial interest in the lens, but it goes further than that. As a result of this lens, I perform very few Nd:YAG capsulotomies, so in fact, the BIL reduces my income from laser treatments and could be considered a financial disinterest. I do not mind this though. The prevention property of the lens is particularly useful in younger patients, diabetics, uveitis patients and children, who are extremely prone to developing PCO. While performing a laser capsulotomy is not difficult in a standard case, young patients or those with mental retardation may not be so simple to laser.

The invention of the anterior capsulorhexis was a great improvement over the previous "can-opener" openings, but the smooth rhexis was also associated with the proliferation of anterior lens epithelial cells (A-LECs) causing contraction; this had not been observed in the previous capsular opening techniques. In its most exaggerated form, it causes extreme reduction and malpositioning of the capsular opening and can cause displacement of the IOL and retinal detachment [5]. Capturing the anterior rhexis in the BIL groove confines the fibrotic changes and mechanically

Table 2.1 Pros and cons of the BIL technique

Pros	Cons
No PCO, cases where Nd:YAG is difficult	Nd:YAG capsulotomy is not difficult
No phimosis	Learning curve
Remains centred	More steps
Does not tend to rotate	Zonular injury
Safe to perform PPCCC	Is PPCCC not risky?
Easy to exchange	
Useful in cases where refractive outcomes are not guaranteed, e.g. keratoconus or post-RKs	

prevents contraction and rhexis phimosis. The fibrotic reaction also tends to be "sticky" and holds the lens in place, and, as a result, the lens remains well-centred [6] and is resistant to rotation [7, 8].

Another interesting feature of the lens design is that there are no haptics in the capsular bag. This makes the lens very simple to disengage from the bag in the event of an explantation. Despite the fact that the posterior capsule has been opened during the PPCCC, exchanging the lens is one of the simplest and easiest lens explantation techniques. This is an advantage in cases for which the refractive outcome is difficult to guarantee. In our centre, we find it particularly useful in cases of keratoconus or post-radial keratotomy where even the best predictive formulae can still result in refractive surprises. In these cases, laser correction of the residual refractive error is difficult; exchanging the lens is the easiest approach in this case.

In the future, we hope to see a multifocal lens version come to market. This would yield the advantage of preventing PCO, which can have a very significant effect on the multifocality of the lenses. It would also allow easy exchange. An overview is provided below (Table 2.1):

2.4 Limitations of the BIL

There must still be some residual capsular support in order to implant a BIL. If there is no capsular bag whatsoever, a BIL should not be implanted, and alternative methods of IOL fixation should be considered. Moreover, the benefits of PCO prevention are not relevant when there is no capsule. The capsular bag support does not have to be perfect though. While both capsulorhexes are preferred, the BIL only requires one capsulorhexis, either anterior or posterior, to support it. So, should one rhexis run out or tear, the lens can still be used.

The implantation of the lens is more complicated than that of a typical lens-in-the-bag, and as a result, there is an associated learning curve. The size and position of the capsulorhexis are key and can be quite unforgiving. Too small a capsulorhexis and the lens will be difficult to implant and will require a bimanual implantation technique or risk damaging the zonular suspension. Too large a rhexis and the lens will be at risk of rotation and dislocation. This can take a number of repetitions before it becomes intuitive. There are also postoperative risks seen with the BIL that do not occur with other implants. The BIL groove can trap the iris postoperatively, and a painful pupil block can occur if the iris becomes completely incarcerated.

2.5 Core Messages

The bag-in-the-lens implant can confer a number of advantages over the standard lens-in-the-bag approach. It is more difficult, however, and it requires a higher degree of technical precision, but when you see the lens in situ, years after the primary implantation, it is very satisfying to see how clear and stable it is.

The aim of this book is to help new BIL users to tap into the experience of established users, to reduce risks and complications and to shorten the learning curve associated with this technique.

References

1. Tassignon MI. Morcher GmbH, assignee. Intraocular lens and method for preventing secondary opacification. US patent 6 027 351 2000.
2. Tassignon M, De Veuster I, Godts D, Kosec D, Van den Dooren K, Gobin L. Bag-in-the-lens intraocular lens implantation in the pediatric eye. J Cataract Refract Surg. 2007;33:611–7.
3. Tassignon M, Gobin L, Mathysen D, Van Looveren J, De Groot V. Clinical outcomes of cataract surgery after bag-in-the-lens intraocular lens implantation following ISO standard 11979-7:2006. J Cataract Refract Surg. 2011;37:2120–9.
4. Leysen I, Coeckelbergh T, Gobin L, Smet H, Daniel Y, DeGroot V, Tassignon MJ. Cumulative neodymium:YAG laser rates after bag-in-the-lens and lens-in-the-bag intraocular lens implantation: comparative study. J Cataract Refract Surg. 2006;32:2085–90.
5. Davison JA. Capsule contraction syndrome. J Cataract Refract Surg. 1993;19:582–9.
6. Verbruggen K, Rozema JJ, Gobin L, Coeckelbergh T, DeGroot V, Tassignon MJ. Intraocular lens centration and visual outcomes after bag-in-the-lens implantation. J Cataract Refract Surg. 2007;33:1267–72.
7. Tassignon M, Gobin L. Toric bag-in-the-lens implant: why and how to implant. Exp Rev Ophthalmol. 2010;5:135–41.
8. Gobin L, Tassignon MJ, Mathysen D. Spherotoric bag-in-the-lens intraocular lens: power calculation and predictive misalignment nomogram. J Cataract Refract Surg. 2011;37:1020–30.

3 Histopathological Aspects of Bag-in-the-Lens Implantation

Liliana Werner

3.1 Introduction

This chapter involves the description of the histopathological features of six human eyes implanted with the foldable, hydrophilic acrylic bag-in-the-lens (BIL), obtained postmortem at different postoperative times from four patients. Pathological analyses confirmed the concept of the BIL design in that residual proliferative/regenerative material remains confined to the intercapsular space of the capsular bag remnant outside the optic rim.

The "bag-in-the-lens" (BIL) concept, developed by Dr. Tassignon in Belgium, completely changes the relationship between the intraocular lens (IOL) and the capsular bag, eliminating the contact between the lens and the inner surface of the latter [1–9]. It involves the use of a twin capsulorhexis lens design and the performance of anterior and posterior capsulorhexes of the same size. When both capsules are well-stretched around the optic of the lens, any remaining lens epithelial cells (LECs) will be captured within the remaining space of the capsular bag, and their proliferation will be limited to this space; in so doing, posterior capsule opacification (PCO) will be prevented. We had the opportunity to receive a series of six human eyes obtained postmortem in our laboratory at the Moran Eye Center, from four patients who received BIL implantation at different time points before their death [10, 11]. This chapter's purpose is to describe the histopathological findings of this series, which helps in providing a better understanding of the effect of BIL implantation on the human eye.

L. Werner (✉)
John A Moran Eye Center, University of Utah, Salt Lake City, UT, USA
e-mail: liliana.werner@hsc.utah.edu

M.-J. Tassignon et al. (eds.), *Innovative Implantation Technique*,
https://doi.org/10.1007/978-3-030-03086-5_3

Table 3.1 Characteristics of the patients included in this analysis

Patient #	Eye #	Age at implantation	Gender	Date of implantation	Date of death	Postoperative time	Cause of death
1	1 (OD)	86	Male	5-Jun-07	12-Oct-07	4 months	Lung cancer
2	2 (OD)	59	Female	13-Apr-06	5-Jul-08	27 months	Breast cancer
3	3 (OD)	66	Female	20-May-05	12-Jul-08	38 months	Ovarian cancer
3	4 (OS)	65	Female	11-Apr-05	12-Jul-08	39 months	Ovarian cancer
4	5 (OD)	86	Female	23-Apr-08	2-Feb-09	9 months	Diabetes type II/ severe aortic valve stenosis
4	6 (OS)	86	Female	23-Apr-08	2-Feb-09	9 months	Diabetes type II/ severe aortic valve stenosis

3.2 Patients

Table 3.1 summarizes the characteristics of the patients included in this analysis. All patients received BIL implantations in Belgium, performed either by Dr. Tassignon or by her associates. For two of the four patients, the implantation of the BIL was performed bilaterally, and so both eyes were analyzed. The patients were aged 74.6 ± 12.6 years at implantation. The postoperative time in this series ranged from 4 to 39 months.

3.3 Surgical Procedure for BIL Implantation

A ring-shaped caliper was used to assist with the anterior capsulorhexis sizing and centration, according to previously described techniques for BIL implantation [8]. Eye numbers 1, 2, and 6 were implanted by a surgeon experienced with BIL implantation, and eye numbers 3 and 4 were implanted by a surgeon who was moderately experienced with BIL implantation at the time of surgery. The procedures for all eyes, save for number 5, were uneventful. The procedure in eye number 5 was initiated by a fellow at the beginning of his learning curve at the time of surgery. During the procedure, the anterior capsulorhexis tore off temporally, and the procedure was completed by an experienced surgeon. BIL implantation was still possible although in a relatively decentered position, given that the posterior capsulorhexis was intact. Clinical BIL decentration was insignificant in all eyes for which the surgical implantation was uneventful postoperatively. In eye number 5, a relative lens decentration was observed postoperatively, but without clinical significance as this was a monofocal, spherical lens. The BIL's special design renders its centration and postoperative stability primarily dependent on the position of the two capsulorhexes, and eye number 5 illustrates this fact well.

3.4 Ultrasound and Macroscopic Analyses of Enucleated Eyes

Upon the patients' deaths, the eyes were enucleated and sent to the John A. Moran Eye Center, University of Utah, for analysis; they were immersed in 10% neutral-buffered formalin. After gross inspection, each eye underwent scanning under a high-frequency ultrasound system (Artemis, Ultralink) to assess BIL centration and fixation. In each case, ultrasound examination revealed the presence of a well-fixated, well-centered IOL located at the level of the capsular bag (Fig. 3.1a) save for eye number 5; the BIL in eye number 5 appeared slightly decentered (Fig. 3.1b).

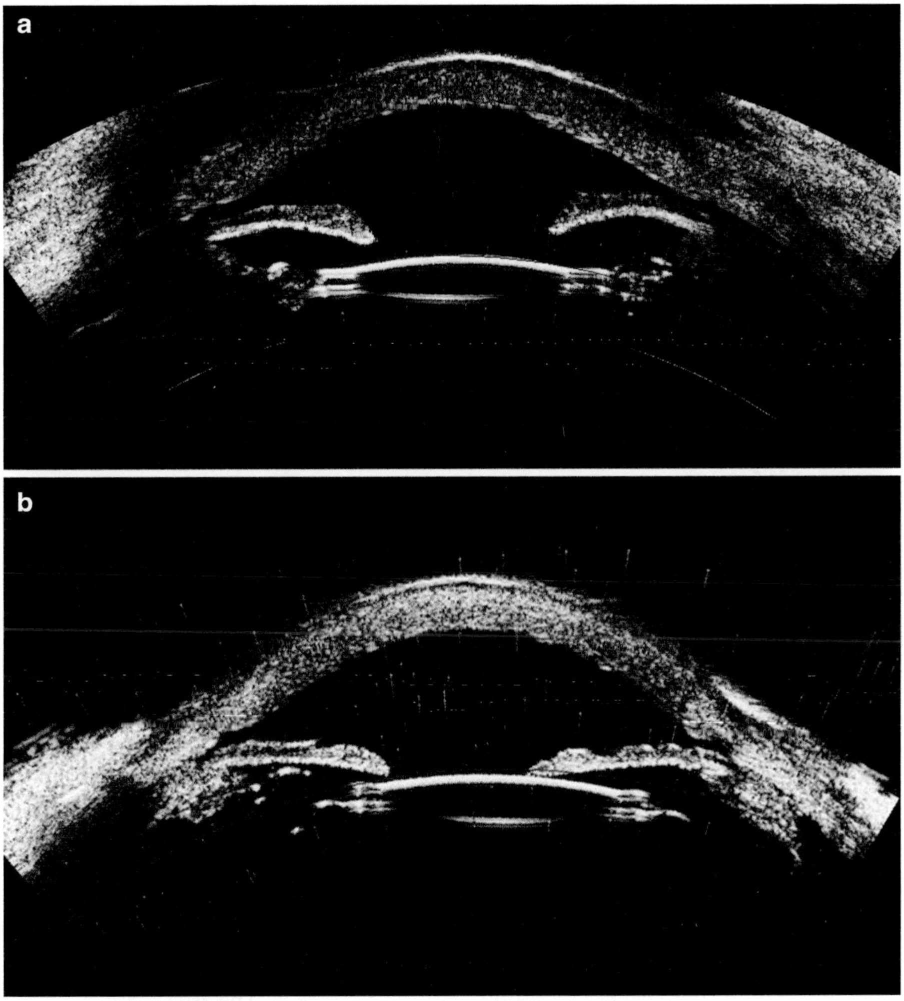

Fig. 3.1 High-frequency ultrasound scans of two of the eyes implanted with the bag-in-the-lens and obtained postmortem. (**a**) Eye #2. (**b**) Eye #5

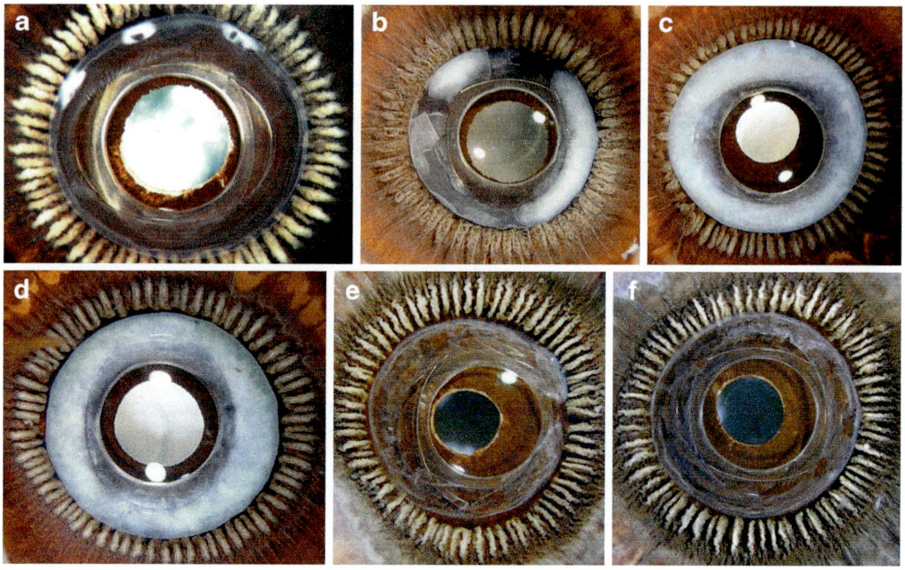

Fig. 3.2 Gross photographs from the posterior or Miyake-Apple view of the six eyes implanted with the bag-in-the-lens and obtained postmortem. (**a–f**) Eye #1 through #6, respectively

Table 3.2 Analyses of the bag-in-the-lens centration[a]

Eye #	Capsular bag diameter	Average space in the periphery of the capsular bag	Decentration in relation to the capsular bag
1	9.52	2.26	0.033
2	9.78	2.39	0.161
3	9.62	2.31	0.301
4	9.71	2.36	0.157
5	9.12	2.06	0.721
6	9.00	2.25	0.166

[a]Quantified with the Matlab 6.5 program (MathWorks). Measurements in mm

Each eye was then sectioned at the equator, and the gross examination of the anterior segment was performed from a posterior or Miyake-Apple view (Fig. 3.2). Gross examination confirmed the presence of the overall circular IOL, with anterior and posterior capsule openings well-stretched around the lens optic. Fibrosis of the rhexis edges was observed, in eye numbers 2–4 more prominently so (postoperative time, 27–39 months). The overall round shape of the capsular bag was maintained in each case, without any distortion or ovalization. The central area delimitated by the rhexis openings remained perfectly clear in all eyes. In eye number 1 (postoperative time, 4 months), three patches of regenerative/proliferative whitish material were observed in the equatorial region of the capsular bag (beginning of Soemmering's ring formation). The capsular bag was otherwise clear. The bag was also mostly clear in eye numbers 5 and 6 (postoperative time, 9 months). More significant Soemmering's ring formation was observed in eye number 2 (postoperative time, 27 months), occupying approximately 1/2 of the periphery of the capsular bag. Abundant Soemmering's ring formation was observed for 360° in the capsular bag of eye numbers 3 and 4 (postoperative time, 38 and 39 months).

Gross photographs were imported into a custom computer program in Matlab 6.5 (MathWorks), for assessment of the BIL centration in relation to the capsular bag periphery done by Dr. Tassignon's group [7]. Circles that were concentric with the capsular bag periphery were projected onto the photographs, and the center of each circle was calculated and marked. An analysis of centration is shown in Table 3.2. As expected, decentration was more observed in eye number 5 (Table 3.2).

3.5 Microscopic (Histopathological) Analyses of Enucleated Eyes

The anterior segment of each eye that contained the BIL was then prepared for histopathological examination, and histopathological sections stained with Masson's trichrome stain were analyzed under an Olympus light microscope. Histopathological sections passing through the center of the capsular bag showed anterior and posterior capsule openings directed to the groove at the periphery of the lens (Fig. 3.3a, b). In this configuration, any regenerative/proliferative material would remain

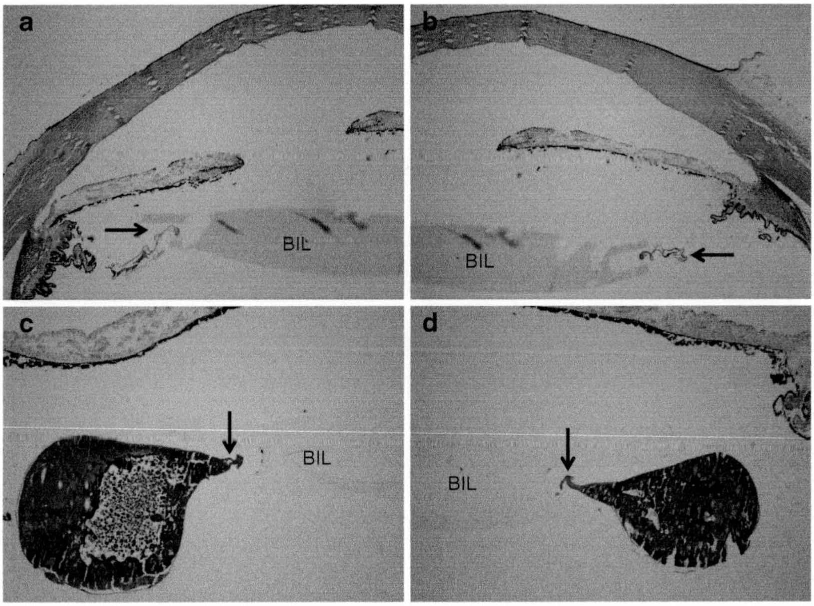

Fig. 3.3 Histopathological sections cut from two of the eyes implanted with the bag-in-the-lens and obtained postmortem. (**a**, **b**) Eye #6. The arrows show anterior and posterior capsules directed to the groove of the bag-in-the-lens (BIL). Masson's trichrome stain; original magnification X20. (**c**, **d**) Eye #3. The arrows show the sites of adhesion between anterior and posterior capsules, mediated by fibrocellular tissue at the inner surface of the anterior capsule. Masson's trichrome stain; original magnification X40

confined to the intercapsular space of the capsular bag remnant outside the optic rim/groove, which was observed in the gross analysis of the eyes and confirmed by histopathological evaluation. Cortical material and pearls were found within the Soemmering's ring formation (Fig. 3.3c, d). A tissue composed of LECs and fibrosis was present on the inner surface of the anterior capsule, apparently mediating adhesion between anterior and posterior capsules at the rhexis sites (more clearly observed in eye numbers 2–4; Fig. 3.3c, d).

3.6 Implications of Histopathological Findings to BIL Implantation

It appears that a fibrocellular tissue developed during the first postoperative year on the inner surface of the anterior rhexis margin (rhexis fibrosis), which mediated adhesion between anterior and posterior capsules at that site, inside the IOL groove (Fig. 3.3c, d). This probably helped to enhance the postoperative stability of the lens and the confinement of any regenerative/proliferative material to the capsular bag's remaining space.

The results described in this chapter confirm previous studies on preclinical studies (in vitro studies using both a human capsular bag model and studies in rabbit eyes) [1, 2, 9], as well as clinical evaluation of the BIL in adult and pediatric eyes [4–8]. BIL implantation was highly effective in preventing PCO in all studies whenever the anterior and posterior capsules were properly secured in the peripheral groove of the IOL.

In conclusion, the evaluation of the postmortem eyes described here, which represent unique specimens, confirmed the BIL concept. The decentration of the lens, in relation to the center of the capsular bag, was insignificant but can be improved by new alignment devices. Any proliferative/regenerative material remains confined to the intercapsular space of the capsular bag remnant outside the optic rim.

References

1. Tassignon MJ, De Groot V, Vrensen GF. Bag-in-the-lens implantation of intraocular lenses. J Cataract Refract Surg. 2002;28:1182–8.
2. De Groot V, Tassignon MJ, Vrensen GF. Effect of bag-in-the-lens implantation on posterior capsule opacification in human donor eyes and rabbit eyes. J Cataract Refract Surg. 2005;31:398–405.
3. Tassignon MJ, De Groot V, Van Tenten Y. Searching the way out for posterior capsule opacification. Verh K Acad Geneeskd Belg. 2005;67:277–88. Review.
4. De Groot V, Leysen I, Neuhann T, Gobin L, Tassignon MJ. One-year follow-up of bag-in-the-lens intraocular lens implantation in 60 eyes. J Cataract Refract Surg. 2006;32:1632–7.
5. Leysen I, Coeckelbergh T, Gobin L, et al. Cumulative neodymium:YAG laser rates after bag-in-the-lens and lens-in-the-bag intraocular lens implantation: comparative study. J Cataract Refract Surg. 2006;32:2085–90.
6. Tassignon MJ, De Veuster I, Godts D, et al. Bag-in-the-lens intraocular lens implantation in the pediatric eye. J Cataract Refract Surg. 2007;33:611–7.

7. Verbruggen KH, Rozema JJ, Gobin L, et al. Intraocular lens centration and visual outcomes after bag-in-the-lens implantation. J Cataract Refract Surg. 2007;33:1267–72.
8. Tassignon MJ, Rozema JJ, Gobin L. Ring-shaped caliper for better anterior capsulorhexis sizing and centration. J Cataract Refract Surg. 2006;32:1253–5.
9. De Keyzer K, Leysen I, Timmermans JP, Tassignon MJ. Lens epithelial cells in an in vitro capsular bag model: lens-in-the-bag versus bag-in-the-lens technique. J Cataract Refract Surg. 2008;34:687–95.
10. Werner L, Tassignon MJ, Gobin L, Rozema J, Davis D, Brubaker J. Bag-in-the-lens: first pathological analysis of a human eye obtained postmortem. J Cataract Refract Surg. 2008;34:2163–5.
11. Werner L, Tassignon MJ, Zaugg BE, De Groot V, Rozema J. Clinical and histopathologic evaluation of six human eyes implanted with the bag-in-the-lens. Ophthalmology. 2010;117:55–62.

The History of the Anterior Interface

4

Marie-José Tassignon

4.1 Introduction

I designed the bag-in-the-lens (BIL) implant based on the anatomical characteristics of the anterior interface. Having been a pupil of Jan Worst (Chap. 1), I assumed that the anterior interface anatomy was well known to everybody, but I was totally wrong. Although the structure and anatomy of the posterior interface are very well known, the anterior interface remains enigmatic for most ophthalmologists. The history of its discovery is very exciting and of paramount importance to fully understand the core of the BIL implantation technique. What is unknown tends to be feared, and this is certainly the case for the retrolenticular space.

Ophthalmologists in training are taught never to touch the posterior capsule, and this message has been given to them in a quite dogmatic way by their tutors. We have all experienced the quick prolapse of the vitreous, as soon as the posterior capsule is accidentally damaged by any inadvertent or inappropriate movement. We also know that its occurrence is often due to anatomical surprises or personal distraction or technical issues. It is difficult to change dogmas, but in the course of my career, I have made progress in convincing colleagues that the retrolenticular space is not a black box to be avoided.

The key point is that a planned capsulorhexis is completely different to an accidental tear. Vitreous prolapse will not occur when the posterior capsule is opened in a surgeon-controlled way, as described elsewhere in this work (Chap. 8). I would like this idea to replace the previously widespread dogma about the oft-eared posterior capsulorhexis.

M.-J. Tassignon (✉)
Department of Ophthalmology, Antwerp University, University Hospital, Edegem, Belgium
e-mail: marie-jose.tassignon@uza.be

M.-J. Tassignon et al. (eds.), *Innovative Implantation Technique*,
https://doi.org/10.1007/978-3-030-03086-5_4

We measured the fluorescein leakage 24 h after cataract surgery in three groups of patients who had uneventful surgeries, with a lens-in-the-bag implantation, a planned PPCCC with a lens-in-the-bag implantation, and a complicated posterior capsule tear with vitreous prolapse and consequent anterior vitrectomy followed by a lens-in-the-bag implantation. The same pattern of fluorescein diffusion was measured in eyes without PPCCC and in eyes with planned PPCCC by using the fluorophotometer. However, as soon as vitreous prolapse occurred in complicated cataract surgery, fluorescein diffusion into the posterior segment of the eye increased dramatically [1]. The destruction of the anterior vitreous is, therefore, the cause of increased interaction between the anterior and posterior segments of the eye. The ocular barriers are functional as long as the anterior hyaloid remains intact.

Thousands of PPCCCs have been performed by many ophthalmologists worldwide. Although the technique has survived since its introduction in 1990 [2], the fear of performing a surgeon-controlled posterior capsulorhexis still remains. Some leading ophthalmologists have claimed that the posterior capsulorhexis is unsafe and have condemned the technique in books, papers, and magazines. But, why is it then recommended in pediatric cataract and even by the same ophthalmologists who claimed that PPCCC was dangerous? Is it not strange that an allegedly unsafe act is actively promoted for children's eyes?

The only way to convince our colleagues is to teach them about the anatomy of the anterior interface, a still-misunderstood structure by most ophthalmologists in the twenty-first century. The anterior interface has a fabulous history. Modern knowledge about this space starts in the seventeenth century, and we are still learning more about it today.

4.2 The Anterior Interface and Related Structures Described in Literature (Seventeenth Century to Twentieth Century)

Table 4.1 provides an overview of the authors involved in the description of the different structures that define the anterior interface or structures that indirectly relate to the anterior interface. I was fortunate enough to have a dear Belgian colleague, Dr. Frans Van de Velde, now living in Boston, who had easy access to the libraries in order to help me in this search. Not all data have been verified nor can they be verified, but most have. I would therefore sincerely like to thank him for his help. Many technical drawings of the anterior interface have been made, but many of them are wrong. Some confusion in terms and even some incorrect references to authors have also been found.

In his thesis "Ueber den Canalis Petiti und ein Ligamentum hyaloideo-capsulare," *Germain Wieger* [8] described a method by which to color the space of Petit using egg white and quicksilver (mercury). He also referred to a French surgeon, *Jean-Louis Petit*, as having discovered the space named after him. This, I believe, was an error. Jean-Louis Petit (1674–1750) was a famous military surgeon who specialized in bone surgery. His name was given to the anatomical area, the "Petit triangle,"

Table 4.1 Chronological summary of named structures of the anterior interface of the eye and related structures

Named structure(s)	Description	Author	Education	Nationality	Chronology
Petit canal	Anterior hyaloid and posterior zonules	François Paufour du Petit	Anatomist Ophthalmologist Surgeon	France Paris	1664–1741 1726 [3]
Zonules (annulus of Zinn)	Lens zonules (peripapillar structure)	Johann Gottfriend Zinn	Anatomist Botanist	Germany Göttingen	1727–1759 1765 [4]
Martegiani's area	Prepapillary vitreous space where the channel of Cloquet begins	Francesco Martegiani	Anatomist	Italy	Estimated 1780–1860 1814 [5]
Cloquet's canal	Canal arteria hyaloidea	Jules Germain Cloquet	Physician Surgeon	France	1790–1883 1825 [6]
Space of Hannover	Interzonular space	Adolph Hannover	Pathologist (cancer cells)	Denmark	1814–1894 1852 [7]
Stilling's duct	Canal arteria hyaloidea	Jakob Stilling	Ophthalmologist	Germany	1842–1915
Wieger ligament	Circular adhesion of the vitreous to the posterior lens capsule of the lens	Germain Wieger	Physician-ophthalmologist	?	? 1883 [8] PhD
Mittendorf dot (?)	Remains of the anterior section of the artery Hyaloid in the posterior capsule of the lens	William Frederick Mittendorf	Ophthalmologist	USA New York	1845–1917
Bergmeister's papilla	Remaining of the posterior section of the artery Hyaloid on the papilla	Otto Bergmeister	Surgeon Ophthalmologist	Austria Vienna	1845–1918 1886 [9]
Berger's space	Circular space behind the posterior capsule of the lens limited by the Wieger ligament	Emil Berger	Anatomist	Austria Graz	1855–1926 1887 [10]
Egger's line	Circular line of adhesion between the vitreous and the posterior lens	Fritz Egger	Internal medicine	Switzerland	1863–1938
Erggelet's space	Space behind Berger's space where the channel of Cloquet begins	Heinrich Erggelet	Ophthalmologist	Germany Göttingen	1883–1969 1914 [11]
Vitreous cisternae of Worst	Cisternal anatomy	Jan Gerben Frans Worst	Ophthalmologist	The Netherlands Groningen	1928–2015 1995 [12]

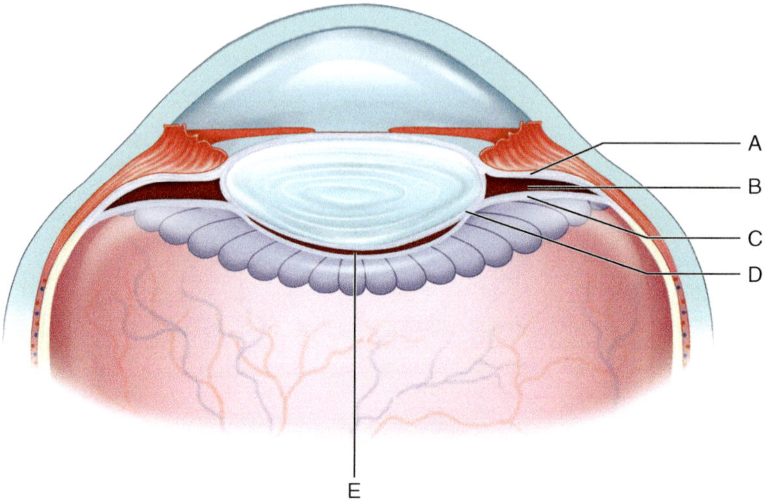

Fig. 4.1 Drawing of the anterior interface as published by Germain Wieger [8]. (**a**) zonules of Zinn, (**b**) Canalis Petiti, (**c**) hyaloid, (**d**) ligamentum hyaloideo-capsulare, (**e**) Fossa patellaris

located at the lumbar area. Jean-Louis Petit was not very interested in the eye, but *François Paufour du Petit* was. This anatomist and ophthalmologist was very much involved with eye diseases. His name was given to an ocular syndrome that describes the opposite features of Horner syndrome. Paufour du Petit, also French and living in Paris, was born in the seventeenth century, the same period as Jean-Louis Petit. In most textbooks, he is considered to have described "Petit canal." The confusion between both in Germain Wieger's book is easily forgiven, given that it is understandable that both scientists could be confused with one another. At that time, all medical doctors were also anatomists, and many structures remained undiscovered.

It is amazing that such a small space, defined as the space between the posterior hyaloid zonule and the anterior hyaloid, was discovered in the seventeenth century. In his thesis, Germain Wieger wrote how happy he was to have been able to demonstrate that Petit was correct in his description of that particular canal. In his drawing, one of the first of its kind (Fig. 4.1), Wieger filled the space behind the posterior capsule with mercury. This area was given the name "fossa patellaris," and he described it as a "lumenlose spatlraum" (empty space). His important contribution was to describe the "ligamentum hyaloideo-capsulare," to which he gave the name "ligamentum." He beautifully described how this structure is made of fibrils (*Streifchen*) that formed a 0.5 mm band. The way Wieger described this ligament was more like a meshwork than a tight band. This is a very important observation, because a ligament will not allow water to pass through, while a meshwork will. Using mercury and egg white, he was incapable of filling the retrolenticular space starting from the Petit canal. The substances he used were too heavy to be able to pass through that ligament.

It would be nice to repeat this anatomical dissection by using dyes of much smaller molecular sizes. This would prove that the Petit canal and the retrolenticular space are in communication with one another. This fluid communication would make a great deal of sense in clinical practice and would explain the hydraulic mechanism of accommodation driven by the ciliary body. This finding, together with the description of *Adolph Hannover's* interzonular canal in 1852 [7], corroborates the hydraulic mechanism. It is obvious that a large amount of aqueous surrounds the crystalline lens, and, therefore, the suggestion that the mechanism of accommodation is based on the displacement of aqueous is easy to make. The role played by the Wieger ligament, and the integrity of its attachment, might be more important regarding accommodation than is currently accepted.

Although Wieger's thesis is very important regarding the knowledge of the anterior interface, I could find neither his date of birth nor the date of his death. His name is often confused with Friedrich Wieger, who wrote textbooks on the history of medicine in 1885 at the University of Strasbourg. It is, therefore, very easy to confuse both scientists. The name "Weigert's ligament" is also described in the literature, which is most probably a typo, transferred from one author to another. The internal medicine doctor, *Fritz Egger* of Switzerland, would later go on to describe the hyaloideo-capsulare adhesion, but the name of Wieger still retains the reference for that particular structure. The lenticular zonules were described by the German anatomist *Johann Gottfriend Zinn* in the eighteenth century. Though his name is more commonly related to the peripapillar annulus of Zinn, it is more commonly related to his second passion, the botanical sciences.

The nineteenth century was rich in anatomical discoveries of the eye. Concerning the anterior interface specifically, the Italian anatomist *Francesco Martegiani* described the peripapillary area of Martegiani in 1814 [5], which will be related to the embryological remnant of the arteria hyaloidea by *Jules Germain Cloquet* in 1825 [6]. Later, the German ophthalmologist *Jakob Stilling* would go on to describe the same canalis hyaloidea, but Cloquet's name remained attached to that structure as the reference. The Austrian surgeon and ophthalmologist *Otto Bergmeister* described in 1886 [9] the pathology regarding the uncomplete resorption of Cloquet's canal at the level of Martegiani's space.

William Frederick Mittendorf (New York, USA) so said described the remnant of the anterior intersection of the arteria hyaloidea with the posterior capsule. This is referred to as the Mittendorf dot. I did, however, not find any confirmation on that description. What we found is that this embryological remnant, is not clinically attached to the posterior capsule, as described in the books. Mittendorf dots are still visible after the bag-in-the-lens implantation, which means that the Mittendorf dot is not attached to the posterior capsule. Ergellet will give us more details about the connection of Mittendorf dot and the Ergellet space (see Chap. 15).

Although the "fossa patellaris" was previously described and colored by Wieger, that space would go on to be related to the name of *Emil Berger*, an Austrian anatomist of the eye. Wieger described the fossa patellaris as a "lumenlose Spaltraume" (empty space), while Emil Berger described it as a real space in his book in 1887 [10]. He specifies that the eye that he dissected and described was from a patient

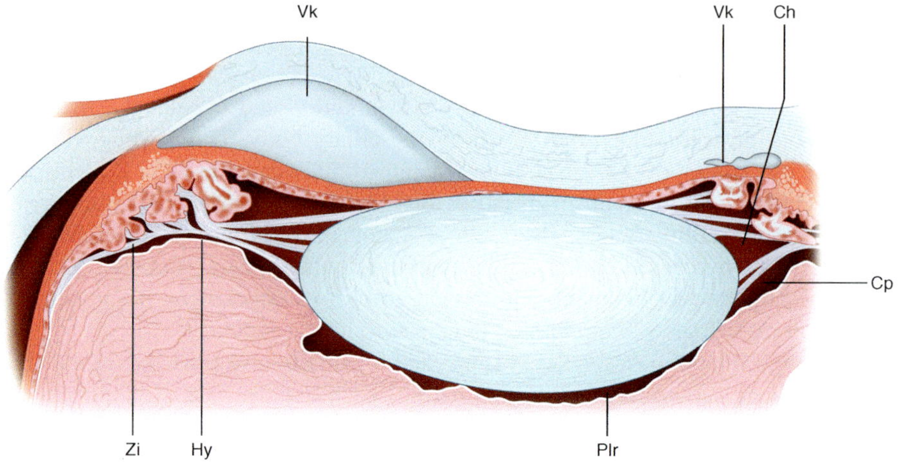

Fig. 4.2 Technical drawing published in Emil Berger's book in 1887 [10]. vk, anterior chamber; ch, canal of Hannover; zi, zonules of Zinn; hy, hyaloid; plr, posterior lenticular space; cp, Petit canal

who presented "uveitis." Iris synechiae with the cornea were, therefore, present on the anatomical section of Fig. 4.2. This is an important detail since it might be that the retrolenticular space, as described by Wieger and Berger, was only visible in pathological conditions. This remains to be examined, but it looks like this space is indeed only visible in aging eyes, high myopes, and eyes with ocular comorbidities, based on our current clinical knowledge and surgical experience. These concepts will be elaborated in greater detail in Chap. 15.

I have not yet discovered who first credited the retrolenticular space to Berger, whose name is now synonymous with this space. I have to return once more to Wieger's work and to his anatomical dissections. He experimentally described how he was capable of detaching the attachments of the ligamentum hyaloideo-capsulare from the posterior capsule. He described the anterior hyaloid detachment in vitro for the first time. Later on, this phenomenon could be observed by several vitreoretinal surgeons, and we were able to describe it peroperatively by means of the OCT [14].

The importance of Fig. 4.3 lies in its correct description of the area behind Berger's space, Erggelet's space. The German ophthalmologist *Heinrich Erggelet* worked closely together with the Swedish ophthalmologist and Nobel Prize winner *Alfred Gullstrand*. Erggelet used Gullstrand's newly invented slit lamp to describe the space behind Berger's space. This space is the anterior equivalent of Martegiani's space. Its attachment is not at the level of the posterior capsule but at the level of the anterior hyaloid, the posterior delineation of Berger's space. This is another very important observation because it assumes that the posterior capsule is left intact in cases of primary fetal proliferation. I looked into these structures very carefully,

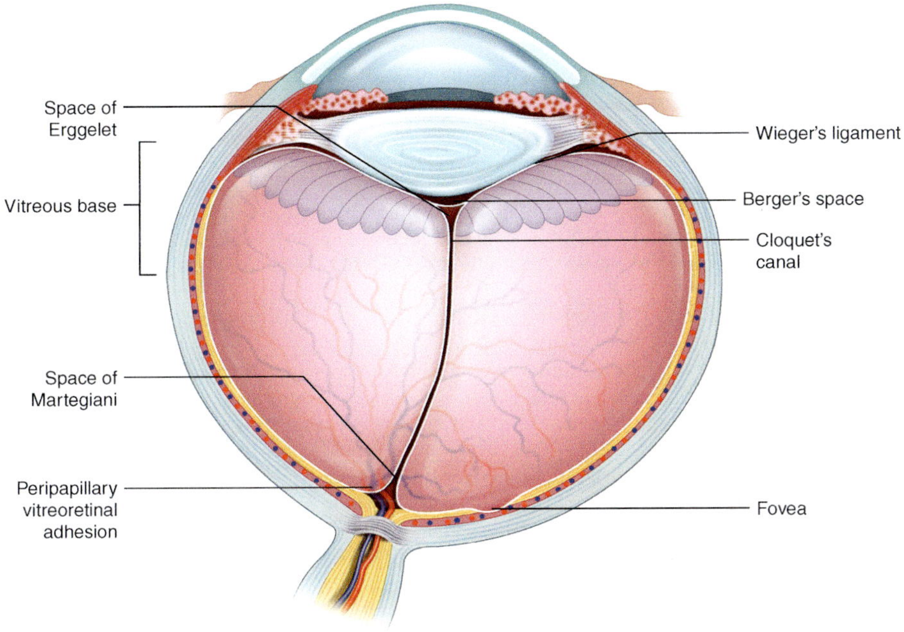

Fig. 4.3 Technical drawing published in a book by Michel RG, Wilkenson CP, and Rice TA [13]

ever since operating on babies with PHPV/PFV. In the few cases that I have operated on, I was able to find the posterior capsule intact and could dissect it from the underlying proliferative and vascularized plaque (video 1, Chap. 15). I can, thus, confirm that Heinrich Erggelet was correct in his description.

More recently, *Jan Worst*, a Dutch ophthalmologist from Groningen, colored Berger's space, using a particular dissection method under water. His book, published in 1995 [12], gives a very thorough historical overview of the anatomy of the vitreous body as a whole.

4.3 Technical Drawings

The three drawings that we have to bear in mind are those by Germain Wieger, Emil Berger, and Michel RG, Wilkenson CP, and Rice TA (Figs. 4.1, 4.2 and 4.3). These three drawings are complementary and describe all of the named structures, as detailed in Table 4.1. They are the most accurate and original drawings that exist. Many drawings of the anterior interface were used thereafter, but many of them are incomplete or wrong.

References

1. De Groot V, Hubert M, Van Best JA, Engelen S, Van Aelst S, Tassignon MJ. Lack of fluorophotometric evidence of aqueous-vitreous barrier disruption after posterior capsulorhexis. J Cataract Refract Surg. 2003;29:2330–8.
2. Gimbel H, Neuhann T. Developments, advantages, and methods of the continuous circular capsulorhexis technique. J Cataract Refract Surg. 1990;16:31–7.
3. François Paufour du Petit « Mémoire de l'Académie des sciences », 1726.
4. Johann Gottfriend Zinn « Descriptio anatomica oculi humani iconibus illustrata », 1765.
5. Francesco Martegiani « Novae Observationes de Oculo Humano » Naples Cajetani Eboli, 1814.
6. Jules Germain Cloquet « Manuel d'anatomie descriptive du corps humain » Paris-Bêchet jeune, 1825.
7. Adolph Hannover « Beiträge zur Anatomie, Physiologie und Pathologie dieses Organs », Leipzig, Editor Leoplod Bols, 1852.
8. Wieger G « Ueber den Canalis Petiti und ein Ligamentum hyaloidea-capsulare ». Heitz. Strassburg, 1883.
9. Otto Bergmeister « Die Intoxicationsamblyopien » Wiener Klinik, 1886.
10. Berger E. Beitrage zur Anantomie des Auges in normalem und pathologischem Zustande. 1st ed. Wiesbaden: JF Bergmann. p. 1887.
11. Heinrich Ergellet "Befunde bei fokaler Beleuchtung mit der Gullstrandschen Nernstspaltlampe. Klin Monatschr Augenheilk 53:II, 1914.
12. Gerben J, Worst F. Cisternal anatomy of the vitreous. Amsterdam/New-York: Kugler Publications; 1995.
13. Michael RG, Wilkenson CP, Rice TA. Retinal detachment. St. Louis: Mosby; 1990.
14. Tassignon MJ, Ni Dhubhghaill S. Real time intraoperative optical coherence tomography imaging confirms older concepts about the Berger space. Ophthalmic Res. 2016;56(4):222–6.

Clinical Variations of the Vitreo-lenticular Interface

5

Marie-José Tassignon

5.1 Introduction

Since the publication of our very first clinical observations about the vitreo-lenticular interface [1] using the per-operative OCT coupled to the Lumera Zeiss microscope, we have systematically recorded and reviewed our clinical cases in order to apply the theoretical knowledge we learned from Chap. 4, entitled "History of the Anterior Interface." It has been a real pleasure for us to look for the named structures of the anterior interface as described by our predecessors and to give them the recognition that they deserve. This chapter ought, therefore, to be considered as a tribute to the scientists of the seventeenth to twentieth centuries who dedicated their time and interest to the anterior interface of the eye.

The interest of the ophthalmologists for the anterior interface began with the introduction of two new surgical techniques: the optic capture and the bag-in-the-lens (BIL). Both techniques have in common that they look behind the posterior capsule. The optic capture technique [2] was initially proposed to equip an eye with an intraocular lens in adverse conditions, including cases of inadvertent posterior capsule rupture or cases with planned PPCCC in combination with an anterior vitrectomy. The BIL technique purposely uses the space of Berger after having performed a surgeon-controlled PPCCC. In the optic capture technique, most of the anatomy of the anterior interface was "cleaned" effectively by means of an anterior vitrectomy,

Electronic Supplementary Material The online version of this chapter (https://doi.org/10.1007/978-3-030-03086-5_5) contains supplementary material, which is available to authorized users.

M.-J. Tassignon (✉)
Department of Ophthalmology, Antwerp University, University Hospital, Edegem, Belgium
e-mail: marie-jose.tassignon@uza.be

M.-J. Tassignon et al. (eds.), *Innovative Implantation Technique*,
https://doi.org/10.1007/978-3-030-03086-5_5

while the BIL technique respects the anatomical integrity of the anterior interface to accommodate both the optic and the posterior haptic of the intraocular lens.

By respecting the anatomical integrity, it was possible to describe the anatomical variations of the anterior interface. Fascinated by the images of the lens capsule, imaged with the real-time OCT of the Lumera Zeiss microscope, the variations in size and shape of the Berger space after cataract surgery became obvious. Fully aware that these real-time OCT images were being taken after the removal of the crystalline lens, meaning that the water column of the phaco machine might have played a role in this; it certainly illustrates the status of the anterior interface as it is after cataract surgery and the eventual implantation of a bag-in-the-lens intraocular lens. The role of these anatomical variations on the final position of the IOL and refractive outcome is unknown at present and should be studied in the near future. Variations in this interface could be one of the causes for hitherto unexplained postoperative refractive surprises.

In order to study the influence of these variations, it would be very useful to visualize the presence of a detached ligament of Wieger preoperatively. Unfortunately, the OCT images acquired with the devices available at present are not of a sufficiently high resolution to perform these studies. When the natural crystalline lens is removed from the capsule bag and replaced by an intraocular lens, the space that becomes free is very important. The crystalline lens typically has a thickness of approximately 4 to 5 mm and is replaced by an artificial IOL with a maximum thickness of 1 mm. Even if we cannot calculate this space with great accuracy, it is not difficult to imagine that the ciliary body will have to compensate this space in one way or another. Figure 5.1 is an attempt to illustrate this phenomenon and gives an approximation of the important changes in volume that occur in the anterior chamber and the retro-lenticular space after cataract surgery. The drawings that will be used in this chapter were all drawn by Rudi Leysen, medical photographer at the department of ophthalmology of the University Hospital of Antwerp between 1994 and 2016.

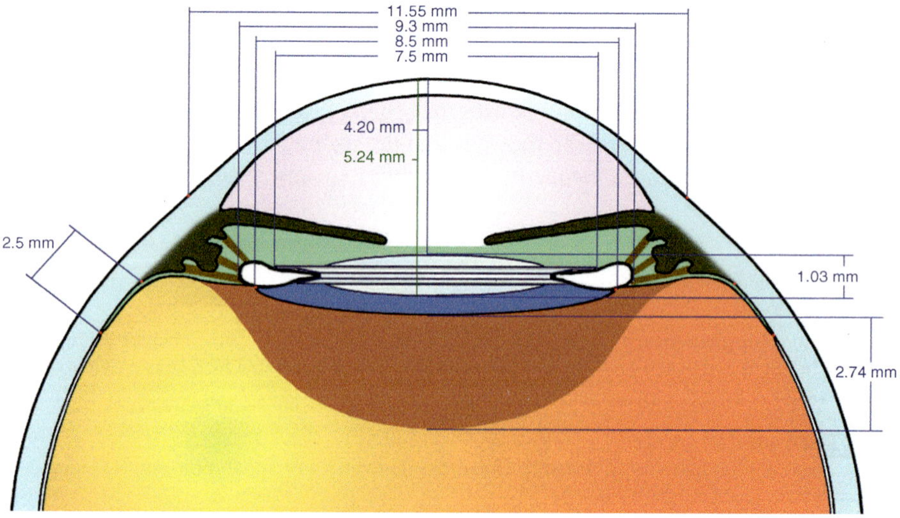

Fig. 5.1 Technical drawing of the anterior interface after cataract surgery and BIL implantation

5.2 Clinical Variations in Anterior Interface as Observed by Perioperative OCT

The OCT images and recordings are all taken at the same surgical step during cataract surgery which takes place just prior to performing the posterior capsule puncture and pushing back the anterior hyaloid by means of the OVD, in short:

- ACCC is performed.
- Crystalline lens is removed from the capsule bag.
- Anterior chamber is filled with OVD.
- Anterior and posterior capsule are positioned on the horizontal plane.
- Capsule bag is collapsed (not filled with OVD).

The images are taken on two meridians within a square corresponding to 6 mm. This choice is justified by the intention to reduce the artifacts and deformation of the scans. The square is then moved to the four cardinal peripheral points, temporal, superior, inferior, and nasal, in order to visualize the area in which the ligament of Wieger separates the space of Petit from the space of Berger. As soon as OVD is injected through the posterior capsule puncture, OCT scans are taken by moving more posteriorly in order to be able to observe the posterior displacement of the anterior hyaloid.

5.3 The Normal Eye

Figure 5.2 illustrates what we can expect in most cases of adult patients with biometrics of emmetropic eyes. The image shows the remnants of the anterior capsule after ACCC has been performed. The anterior and posterior capsules are positioned horizontally by

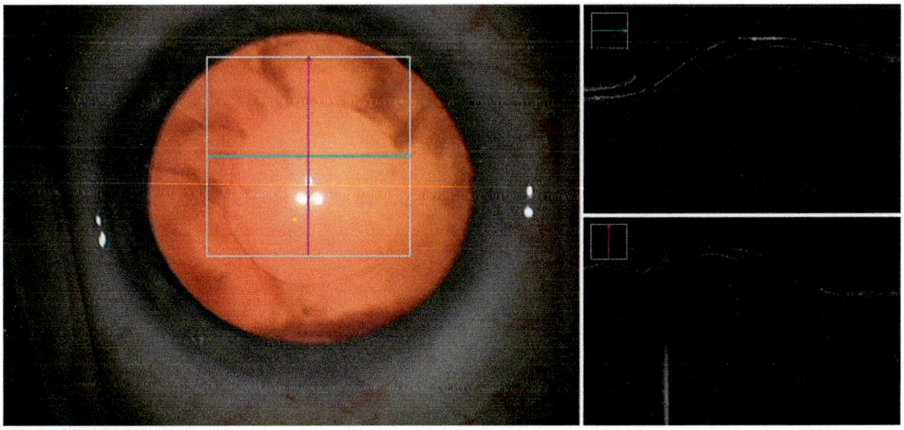

Fig. 5.2 OCT of an adult eye with biometrical parameters within the normal range. The OCT images on the right illustrate the anterior capsule after ACCC, the posterior capsule, and the anterior hyaloid just behind the posterior capsule

means of the OVD injected into the anterior chamber and counteract the positive pressure of the vitreous. The OCT images show the scans of the horizontal and vertical meridian. The videos of that same patient beautifully show the ligament of Wieger separating the space of Petit from the space of Berger while moving the scanner (Video 5.1) and how the anterior hyaloid is pushed posteriorly while OVD is injected through the posterior capsule puncture (Video 5.2). When looking back at Fig. 5.1, we can assume that the anterior hyaloid is in fact positioned back to its original place by the OVD.

5.4 The Myopic Eye and Aging Eye

Figure 5.3 illustrates what we might expect in myopic eyes. Prior to both puncturing the posterior capsule and to injecting the OVD, the anterior hyaloid is located far behind the posterior capsule. The scan is taken at the inferior side of the eye. One can easily imagine that the anterior hyaloid will not touch the posterior capsule at any point. It might reach the posterior hyaloidal zonule or the vitreous base, but this cannot be illustrated because of the iris' blocking effect. This condition is called an anterior vitreous (hyaloid membrane) detachment or AVD and is to be considered the anterior equivalent of the posterior vitreous detachment (PVD). The technical drawing in Fig. 5.4 shows what is considered to be an AVD.

Four clinical signs are very suggestive of AVD:

1. While injecting the OVD through the posterior capsule puncture, the OVD presents a spaghetti-like dispersion into the retro-lenticular space. We cannot speak about the Berger space when the ligament of Wieger is detached. In the case of detachment of the ligament of Wieger, the space of Petit and the space of Berger form one big space: the retro-lenticular space. Video 5.3 shows the spaghetti-like filling of the retro-lenticular space very well.
2. The presence of lens material behind the posterior capsule. Video 5.3 also shows how a small lens debris is present behind the posterior capsule and is pushed

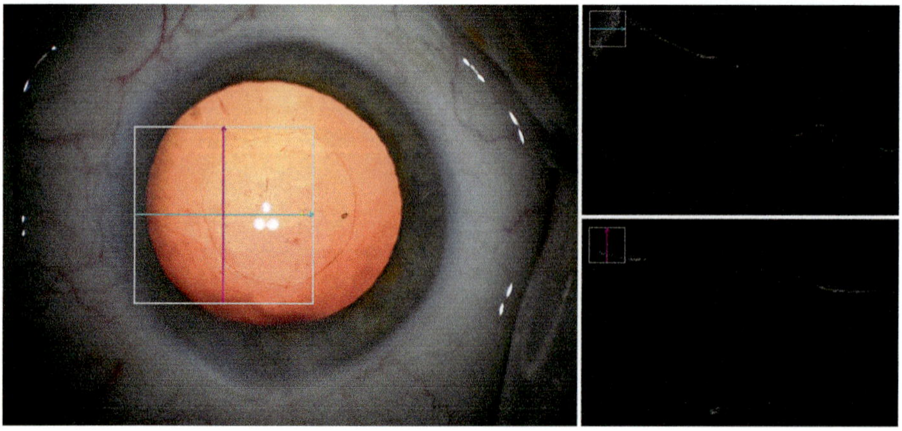

Fig. 5.3 OCT of an adult eye with biometrical parameters of a high myope

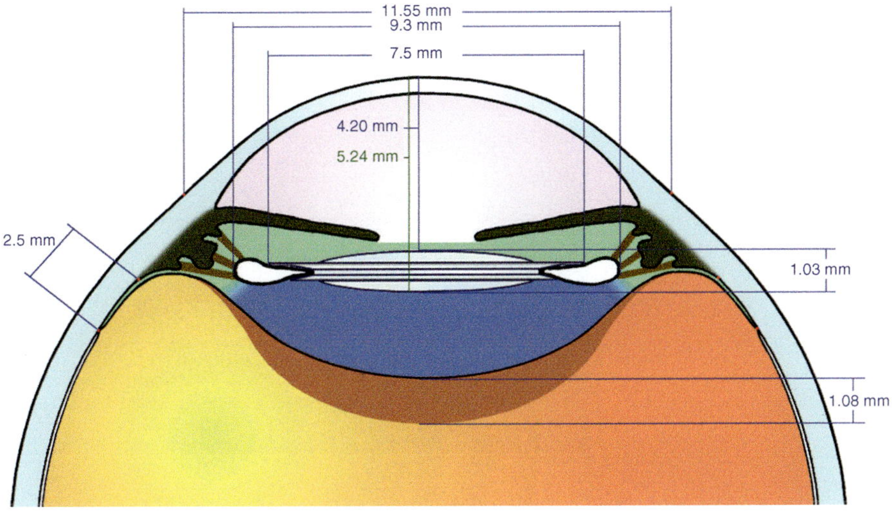

Fig. 5.4 Technical drawing of a complete detachment of the anterior hyaloid after cataract surgery and BIL implantation

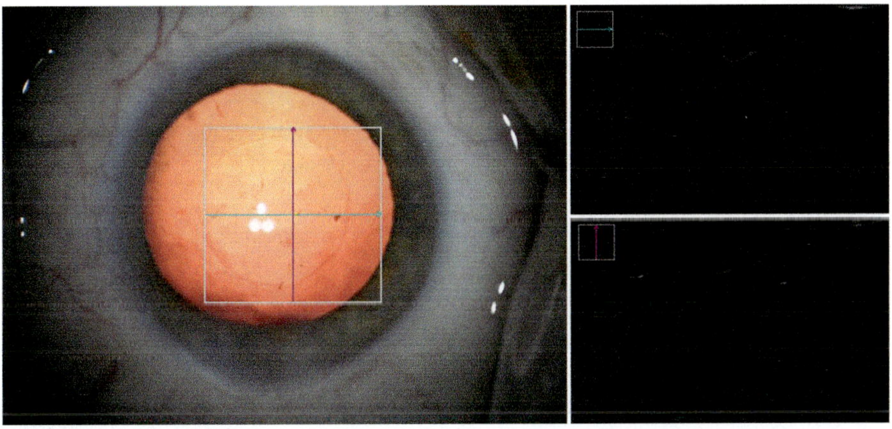

Fig. 5.5 OCT of an adult myopic eye presenting anterior hyaloid detachment and folds in posterior capsule. When folds are observed after removal of the crystalline lens content, this is quite suggestive for AVD

back by the OVD injection. Video 5.4 shows AVD and lens material in this space. These lens fragments have reached this retro-lenticular space through the zonules (most probably). It is impossible to visualize how much these zonules have been damaged with the currently available imaging techniques.

3. When performing irrigation-aspiration in an eye with AVD, the posterior capsule is more easily snapped into the aspiration opening of the IA probe. This can be explained by the increased mobility of the posterior capsule because of the absence of the support through the attachment to the vitreous by the ligament of Wieger. This is illustrated in Fig. 5.5 in which the posterior capsule is completely detached from

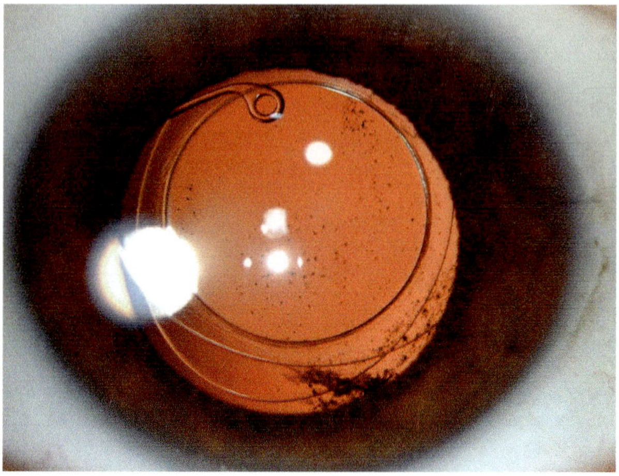

Fig. 5.6 Postoperative anterior segment image of a posttraumatic AVD where a large number of pigment deposits are found on the anterior vitreous hyaloid

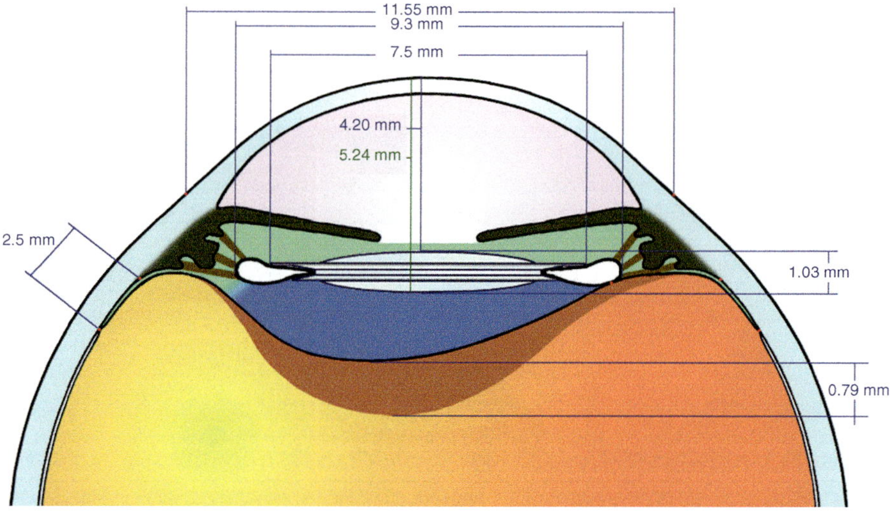

Fig. 5.7 Technical drawing of a partial detachment of the anterior hyaloid after cataract surgery and BIL implantation

the anterior hyaloid and shows many folds. Video 5.5 shows an eye of an aged person presenting with IFIS (stabilized by a Malyugin ring), AVD, and multiple periods where the posterior capsule is snapped into the IA probe. It is evident that this might easily cause posterior capsule rent in unexperienced hands during surgery.

4. The presence of pigment or deposits on the anterior hyaloid, behind the posterior capsule. Figure 5.6 is a postoperative illustration of a posttraumatic AVD with lots of pigment deposits on the anterior hyaloid.

The anterior hyaloid can also be partially detached. Figure 5.7 is a technical drawing illustrating partial anterior vitreous detachment (PAVD). Video 5.6 is a beautiful real-time OCT recording of a PAVD.

5.5 Egger's Line

In Chap. 5, Egger described the line separating the space of Petit and the space of Berger; it can be easily recognized clinically in the instance of pigment deposits in the angle formed by the space of Petit and the ligament of Wieger as shown in Fig. 5.8 and on Video 5.7. Egger's line is pushed back by the OVD injected in the retro-lenticular space because of the complete detachment of the ligament of Wieger.

5.6 Mittendorf Dots

Figure 5.9 shows the Mittendorf dot still present behind the bag-in-the-lens. William Mittendorf was considered the author of this dot (not confirmed though) being the remaining of the anterior section of the arteria hyaloidea and the posterior capsule. The image in Fig. 5.9 contradicts this description. Mittendorf dots are not attached

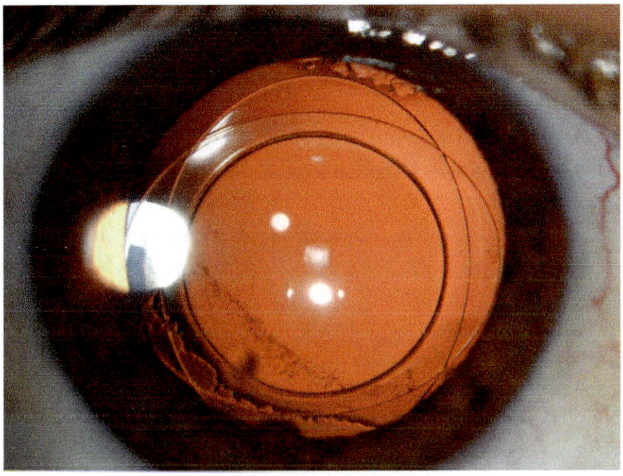

Fig. 5.8 Anterior segment image of a postoperative well-centered bag-in-the-lens implantation and the Egger's line present at the temporal-inferior quadrant behind the lens

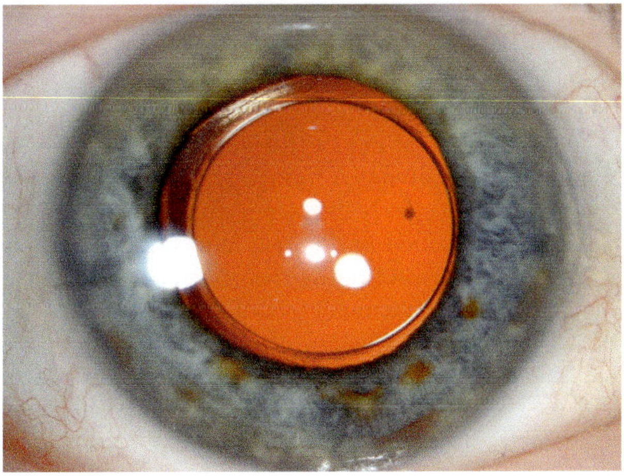

Fig. 5.9 Anterior segment image of a Mittendorf spot still present after implantation of the bag-in-the-lens

to the posterior capsule. They must be attached at the level of the anterior hyaloid. Video 5.8 gives more insights into the relationship of these different structures. It shows the Ergellet space between the Berger space and the Mittendorf dot.

5.7 Erggelet Space

Video 5.8 also shows the Erggelet space. The simultaneous presence of a Mittendorf dot and the Erggelet space in the same patient is a rare and unique finding. The Erggelet space is shown on this video to be attached to the anterior hyaloid. This space is anteriorly located compared to the Mittendorf dot. This observation proves that the Mittendorf dot is certainly not attached to the posterior capsule as described previously in textbooks. Because the Mittendorf dot is clearly located behind the anterior hyaloid and even further away from Erggelet space, this is very suggestive that the Mittendorf dot is the remaining of the arteria hyaloidea with the intersection of the Erggelet space. This hypothesis makes more sense since the Erggelet space is an embryologic remnant of the Cloquet canal as is the Mittendorf dot. This is a new description of the embryological arteria hyaloidea located in Cloquet's canal that ends anteriorly in Erggelet space and posteriorly in Martegiani's space.

5.8 Vitreo-lenticular Interface in Children

The bag-in-the-lens concept yields very beautiful results in congenital, metabolic, and developmental cataract based on a dysgenesis of the anterior interface (Fig. 5.11). By staining the posterior capsule in children who present with an anterior interface dysgenesis (Video 5.9), Van Looveren (staff member of the University Hospital of Antwerp between 2001 and May 2018) was able to demonstrate that repair of this dysgenesis was triggered by cells of mesenchymal origin [3]. The anterior interface is not well developed in these eyes. The anterior hyaloid and the posterior capsule merge at the level of the plaque formation in an attempt to restore the integrity of the posterior lens capsule. This image is completely different from eyes presenting PHPV where the posterior capsule can be dissected from the fibrovascular tissue and is thus intact. PHPV finds its origin at the level of the tunica vasculosa surrounding Cloquet's canal, while in AVLID the pathology is due to the incomplete differentiation of the anterior hyaloid and the posterior capsule.

When looking at the OCT video recordings of eyes that present a subcapsular posterior plaque of toxic origin (Video 5.10), it is evident that in these eyes the posterior capsule is clearly differentiated.

In the publication of the long-term results after bag-in-the-lens implantation in children, Dr Jan Van Looveren observed a very low incidence of visual reproliferation [4]. It was challenging to understand why this might happen. When looking at the OCT images and videos of children, it became obvious that in some children, the Berger space was not big enough to accommodate the bag-in-the-lens properly. Video 5.11 shows the small Berger space in a child eye, which was operated on for congenital cataract. Anterior and posterior capsulorhexes were performed as usual,

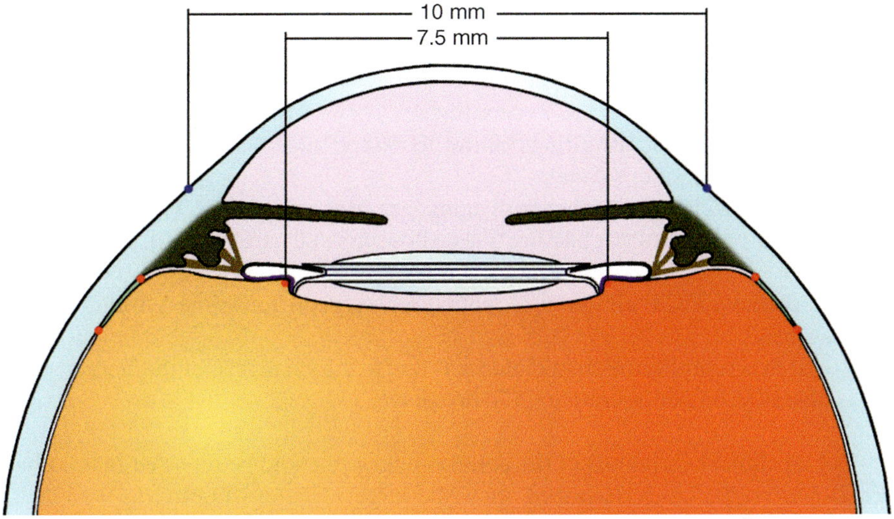

Fig. 5.10 Technical drawing of a small Berger space in a child eye

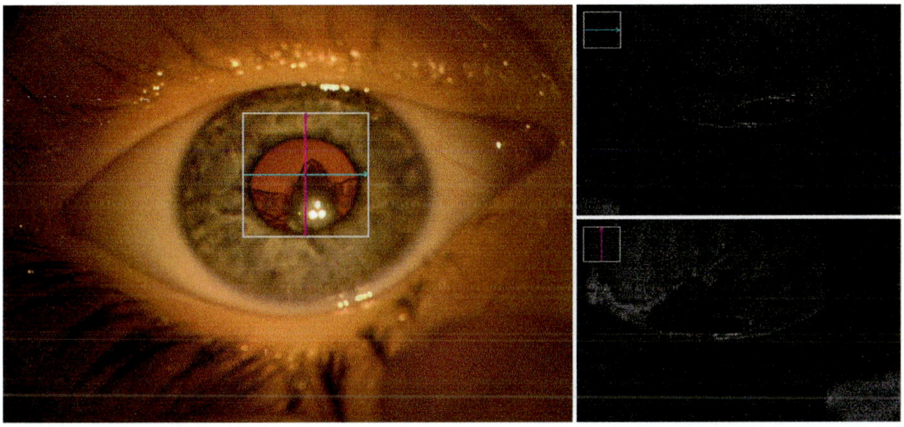

Fig. 5.11 Preoperative scan of a posterior capsule cataract in a child eye. The scan following the pink arrow shows the anterior interface dysgenesis. The posterior capsule appears as interrupted

but the size of the Berger space was not much larger than 6.5 mm in diameter. When inserting a bag-in-the-lens of 7.5 mm in total diameter, this will result in pushing back the posterior capsule by the posterior lens haptic out of the lens groove as shown on the technical drawing (Fig. 5.10). This observation becomes evident when comparing a video of a child with a small Berger space (Video 5.11) with that of an eye with a normal Berger space (Video 5.12). We thus developed a technique to enlarge the Berger space at the desired total diameter in order to correctly accommodate the BIL IOL and avoiding posterior visual axis reproliferation.

5.9 Conclusions

- After cataract surgery, the ligament of Wieger can be found detached, partially or totally, on per-operative OCT recordings.
- Per-operative OCT recordings allow to better understand the embryological structures of Cloquet's canal.
- Berger space changes in size with aging, as observed with OCT per-operatively.
- Acquired subcapsular opacifications show normal structure of the posterior capsule.
- Per-operative OCT allows the ophthalmic surgeon to define vitreo-lenticular dysgenesis
- Visual axis reproliferation in children is due to the small size of the Berger space, as observed on per-operative OCT images.

Not all clinical variations of the anterior interface could be reported in this chapter. However, the cases described show the large variations in size, as well as the large variations in the relation between anterior hyaloid and posterior lens capsule. It is evident that these variations must be fully understood before performing PPCCC using femtosecond laser or any other automated laser device. Not respecting these variations might compromise the physiology of the anterior interface.

References

1. Tassignon MJ, Ni Dhubhghaill S. Real time intraoperative optical coherence tomography imaging confirms older concepts about the Berger space. Ophthalmic Res. 2016;56(4):222–6.
2. Gimbel HV, DeBroff BM. Intraocular lens optic capture. J Cataract Refract Surg. 2004;30(1):200–6.
3. Van Looveren J, Van Gerwen V, Timmermans JP, Tassignon MJ. Immunohistochemical characteristics of the vitreolenticular interface in congenital cataract. J Cataract Refract Surg. 2016;42:1037–45.
4. Van Looveren J, Ní Dhubhghaill S, Godts D, Bakker E, De Veuster I, Mathysen DGP, Tassignon MJ. Pediatric bag-in-the-lens intraocular lens implantation: long-term follow-up. J Cataract Refract Surg. 2015;41(8):1685–92.

Part II

BIL Cataract Surgery

Technical Specifications of the Bag-in-the-Lens Implant

6

Laure Gobin, Sorcha Ní Dhubhghaill, and Marie-José Tassignon

6.1 Introduction

Marie-José Tassignon implanted the first patient with her patented implant in December 1999, the same month I (Laure Gobin) joined her ophthalmology department at the University Hospital of Antwerp. A large part of my job was to coordinate the studies and trials of the implant. The most common long-term complication of modern cataract surgery is posterior capsular opacification (PCO), also known as secondary cataract [1–3]. This process is due to proliferation and migration of residual lens epithelial cells in the capsular bag over the visual axis [4, 5], resulting in opacification and contraction leading to loss of visual acuity [6, 7].

Opening the posterior capsule using an Nd:Yag laser is the most effective treatment for PCO [8]. While this is associated with a low risk of complications [9], it does represent a cost in both time and money to health systems. Meticulous surgical technique including cleaning the capsular bag, covering the edge of the optic with the anterior capsulorhexis, perfect lens positioning, and posterior capsular rhexis can all reduce the risk of PCO but cannot eliminate it completely. Primary posterior capsulorhexis has been shown by De Groot et al. [10] to be prone to cell migration on the posterior face of the IOL or the anterior face of the anterior hyaloid, even in the absence of a posterior capsule. Changes in the implant shape [11–14] (e.g., square edges), changes in implant material, use of antibodies and of special coatings, and the use of a capsular tension ring have all been successful in reducing the proliferation of lens epithelial cells to a degree. There is, however, no surgical approach [15] or lens implant design that is completely successful in eradicating

L. Gobin
Department of Ophthalmology, University Hospital Antwerp, Edegem, Belgium

S. Ní Dhubhghaill · M.-J. Tassignon (✉)
Department of Ophthalmology, Antwerp University, University Hospital, Edegem, Belgium
e-mail: marie-jose.tassignon@uza.be

M.-J. Tassignon et al. (eds.), *Innovative Implantation Technique*,
https://doi.org/10.1007/978-3-030-03086-5_6

PCO, particularly in complicated patients such as children, diabetics, or patients with uveitis [16, 17].

In this chapter, we present the technical specifications of an alternative approach to eliminate PCO called the "bag-in-the-lens" BIL implant [18, 19]. The implant consists of a central optic, similar to other lens implant, but a very different haptic design that not only eradicates PCO but also ensures lens centration. The BIL implant features a central groove that is defined by both the anterior and posterior flanges of the haptics into which the anterior and posterior capsules are inserted. The implantation of this lens requires both anterior and posterior capsules for support so that both anterior and posterior rhexes are required. If the anterior and posterior capsules are properly stretched and captured in the groove, then the epithelial cells will only be able to proliferate in the restricted volume allowed to them [20]. So far, this is the only IOL that can claim to eradicate PCO and provide surgeon-controlled centration, a feature that may become used more frequently in the future.

6.2 Description of the Implant

This BIL implant is a biconvex lens and consists of a central optical zone of 5 mm, and its peripheral haptic design is comprised of two oval elliptical haptics, one anterior and the other posterior. The anterior flange is oval (face) and is oriented perpendicular (90°) to the major axis of the oval of the posterior flange (Fig. 6.1) [19]. The

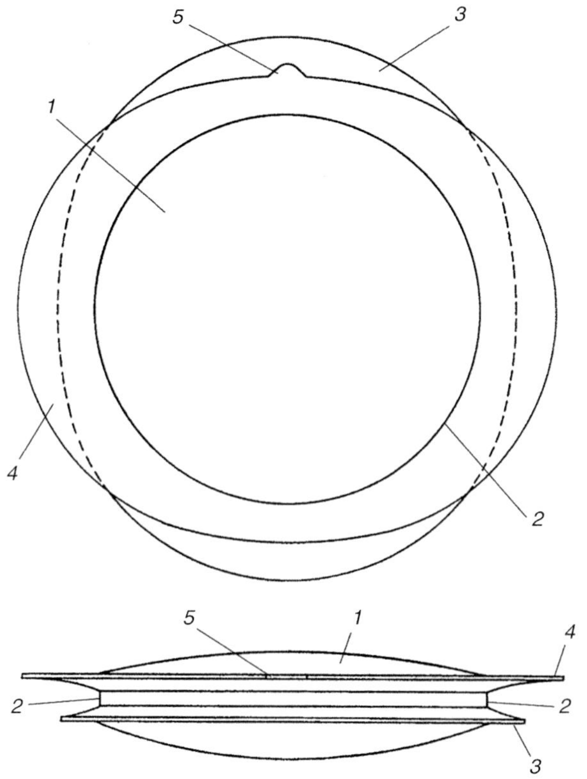

Fig. 6.1 Diagram of the double rhexis implant, illustrating the central optical part surrounded by its haptic. The two oval-shaped anterior and posterior haptics are oriented perpendicular to each other to ensure optimal IOL stability. The side view of the implant shows the characteristic groove in which the two capsules will be placed (1. optic, 2. groove, 3. posterior haptic, 4. anterior haptic, 5. mark of orientation)

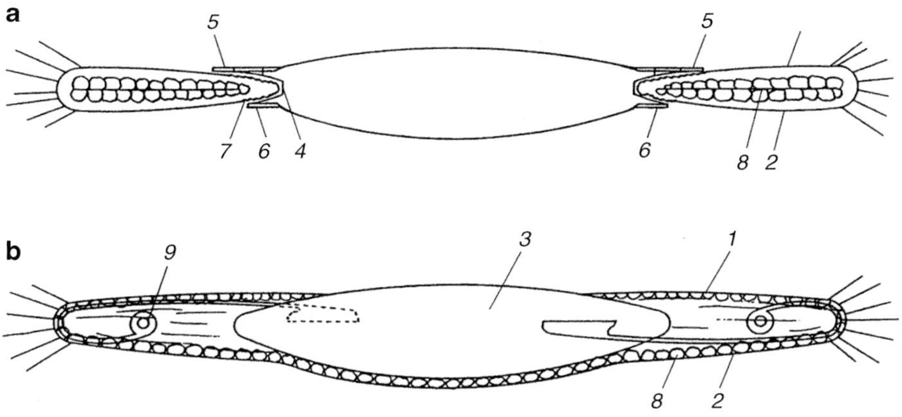

Fig. 6.2 (**a**) "Bag-in-the-lens" lens implant positioned in the double rhexis, where the epithelial cells of the lens are captured in the peripheral portion of the remaining capsule and therefore cannot migrate to the pupillary axis. (**b**) Conventional implantation scheme of the lens in the capsular bag "in-the-bag" showing the epithelial cells of the lens in the equatorial region and on the posterior capsule

shape and orientation of the two haptics have been specifically designed to prevent the tilt of the implant once it has been properly placed (Fig. 6.2a). The first BIL design was made by PhySiol (Belgium), and was a rigid IOL made of PMMA. It was implanted in postmortem donor eyes and living rabbits [20]. Because of excellent results regarding visual axis reproliferation also in rabbits, we decided to convert to a foldable IOL design for the purpose of human implatation. The current implant design (Morcher® 89A, Morcher®, Germany) is made of foldable hydrophilic acrylic material with a water content of approximately 28%. At its widest, the diameter of the implant is 7.5 mm, and at its smallest it is 6.5 mm. Each haptic blade is 0.25 mm with a 0.2 mm groove in between them. This results in a total haptic thickness of 0.6 mm.

6.3 One-Year Follow-Up of the First BIL Implants in 60 Eyes and the Learning Curve

Over 10 years ago, the ethics committee of the University Hospital of Antwerp and AAM-Augenklinik am Marienplatz in Munich approved the use of the BIL implant [21]. The 89A Morcher lens was implanted in 63 eyes of 55 patients presenting cataract with ages ranging from 7 months to 88 years of age (mean 60 years ±25 years). Six children (10 eyes) were included in the cohort, and one child had persistent primary hyperplastic vitreous (PPHV). Preoperatively, the best corrected visual acuity (BCVA) was 0.41 ± 0.23 decimal Snellen. The surgical technique itself is covered in other chapters throughout this book. All patients were examined postoperatively at day 1, day 7, 1 month, 6 months, and 1 year postoperatively.

During the postoperative slit lamp examination, we specifically focused on possible inflammatory reactions, iris configuration, IOL centering, and the proliferation of lens epithelial cells over the optical axis. Dilated fundus examination and an intraocular pressure measurement were performed at every consultation, and slit lamp photos were taken every 6 months. Fluorescein angiography was only performed when macular edema was suspected.

The IOL was implanted in 61 of the 63 patients with no intraoperative complication such as vitreous prolapse. In two cases, however, the capsulorhexis was too small (<4.5 mm in diameter), and the lens could not be squeezed into the opening. At this point in the learning curve, the ring-shaped caliper had not yet been invented. In these cases, the lens was explanted, and a traditional lens was inserted into the capsular bag. The postoperative inflammation was comparable to that induced by the IOLs placed in the capsular bag. No tilt of the lens was observed at the slit lamp or on aberrometry. Two types of complications were observed:

1. Iris capture in the groove of the IOL was observed in three eyes and required surgical correction. After this complication was detected, the surgical procedure was adapted to include a pupil constrictor (Michiol® or Miostat®) at the end of surgery, suturing the corneal incision and using pilocarpine in the early postoperative period. The lens groove was then reduced from 0.4 mm to 0.2 mm, and the haptic flanges were reduced from 0.25 mm to 0.2 mm in thickness.
2. In the case of one child, the rhexis was too large and the IOL dislocated postoperatively in the vitreous. By performing a vitrectomy, the IOL could be removed through the pupil and corneal incision and replaced with an intraocular implant fixed in the sulcus. Since then, a calibration ring (Morcher® Germany, 67-PS1) has been used routinely, and the risk of under- or oversizing of capsular rhexis has been significantly reduced [22].

In the 61 eyes that had no operative issues or complications, the average postoperative follow-up was 22.7 months (range 12–68 months). The BCVA in the 29 adult eyes with senile cataract was 1.02 ± 0.2 D. In 24 patients, the mean difference between the expected refraction calculated with a constant A of 119.0 and the refraction obtained was −0.51 ± 0.82 diopters. Based on data from 58 healthy eyes operated on since and with corrected postoperative visual acuity of at least 0.8 and postoperative follow-up of at least 6 months, the A constant was subsequently recalculated as 118.0–118.2.

The visual axis remained extremely clear in all eyes, even in those of children. Moderate proliferation of lens epithelial cells is present in the periphery of the capsular bag. No fibrosis or wrinkling of the remaining capsular sac was observed except at the junction between the anterior and posterior capsules (Soemmering area).

6.4 Interim Analysis of the Rate Pupil Area Opacification

We compared the occurrence of opacification in the pupillary area with the Morcher® 89A implant to that of a conventional Morcher® 92S implant from the same manufacturer [23]. Both implants are made of the same biomaterial and

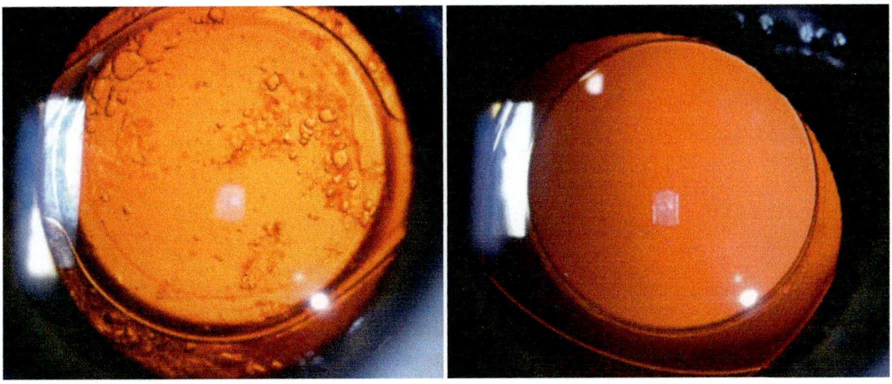

Fig. 6.3 Photos of the two eyes of a 62-year-old patient, 3 years after bilateral cataract. The right eye was implanted with a double rhexis lens (Morcher 89A), while the left eye was implanted with a conventional lens of the same material (Morcher 92S). The difference in transparency is evident between the two eyes. Both lenses are centered; pupil dilation of the right eye was asymmetrical at the time of photography only

differ only in its haptics [24]. The term "opacification of the pupillary area" (OPA) was preferred to "posterior capsular opacification" (PCO) since the posterior capsule is no longer present after implantation of the BIL. The study consisted of a retrospective analysis of the medical records of 181 patients who were operated on using phacoemulsification cataract surgery. Patients received the IOL 92S in one eye and an 89A in the other (Fig. 6.3). Patients were seen postoperatively at day 1, week 1, 5 weeks, 6 months and 1 year after surgery. Laser capsulotomy was performed if there was detectable visual axis opacification and the vision had dropped by at least two lines.

Descriptive statistics (mean, standard deviation, maximum, minimum) were calculated for age, postoperative follow-up, IOL power, and interval between surgery and capsulotomy. Preoperative and postoperative mean visual acuity after 6 months of both groups for patients with no comorbidity (diabetic retinopathy, age-related macular degeneration, etc.), as well as visual acuity before and after capsulotomy are compared. The significance level of the statistical tests was set at 5% (Pearson coefficient value of 0.05). We compared the opacification rates of the two groups by a survival analysis before Nd:YAG laser capsulotomy using the Kaplan-Meier method. Nd:YAG laser capsulotomy was performed in 20% of the eyes of the control group after an average of 20 ± 8 months (9 months to 40 months) after cataract surgery. No capsulotomy was performed in the BIL group. Cumulative capsulotomy incidence rates derived from Kaplan-Meier survival curves were 2% after 1 year and 28.23% after 5.9 years in the 4-year plateau "lens-in-the-bag" group. The cumulative incidence of capsulotomy with the BIL implant was 0% after 6 years. These curves show that after 6 years the OPA probability is 28 times higher with the 92S lens than with the 89A lens [24] (Fig. 6.4).

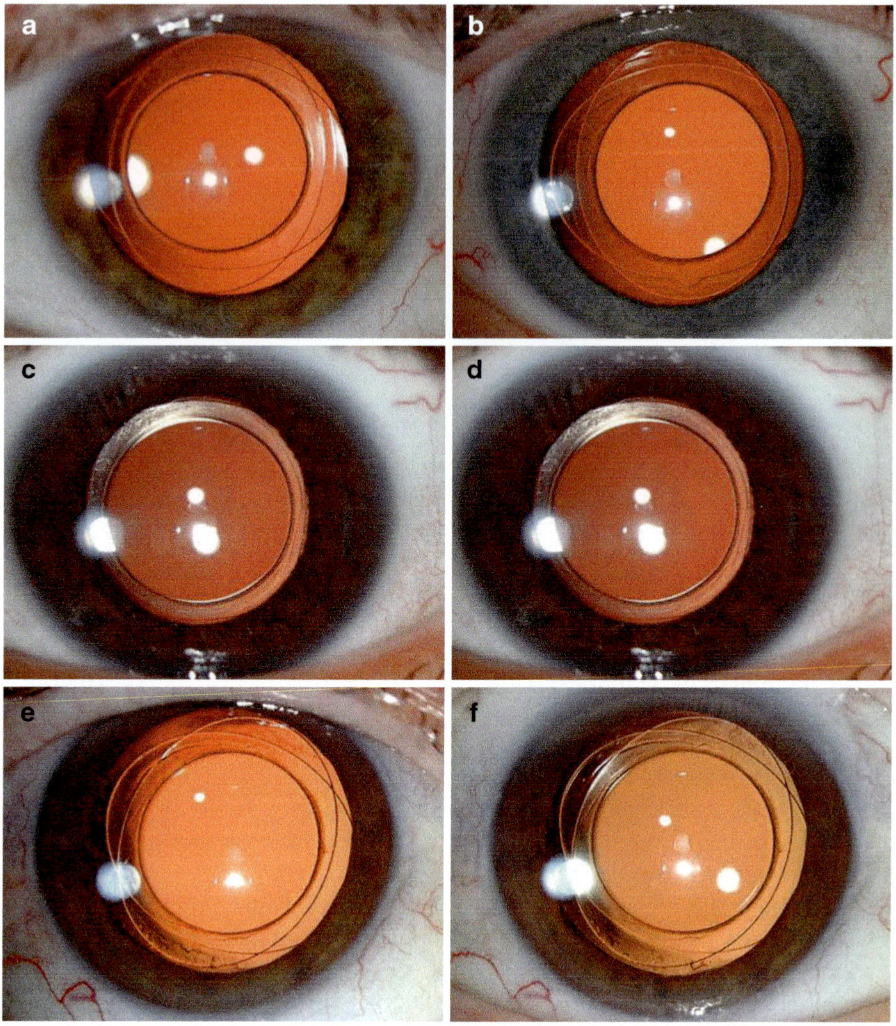

Fig. 6.4 Postoperative photograph of implanted IOL 89A (after (**a**) 6 months, (**b**) 12 months, (**c**) 18 months, (**d**) 24 months, (**e**) 30 months, (**f**) 36 months)

6.5 Analysis of the Postoperative Complications

We followed a cohort of 806 eyes of the first 550 consecutive patients implanted with the "bag-in-the-lens" intraocular lens, between December 2000 and September 2006, without any exclusions. This cohort was followed until January 2010 and involved the application of guidelines of the ISO 11979-6: 2006 standards [25]. Three hundred and twenty-eight eyes in this cohort had serious ocular comorbidities (glaucoma, macular degeneration, etc.). The yearly number of surgeries is shown

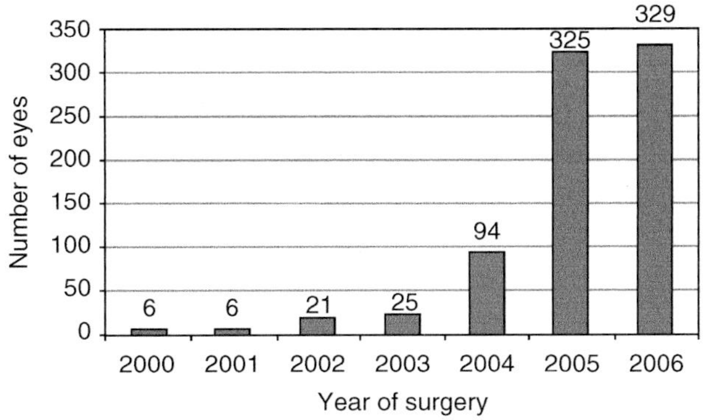

Fig. 6.5 Histogram of BIL implantations between December 2000 and September 2006

Table 6.1 List of adverse effects of the ISO standard: comparison of the occurrence rates of each effect in our cohort compared to the threshold recommended in the standard

	Morcher 89A	Thresholds given by the ISO standard
Temporary		
Cystoid macular edema	0.1% (1/806)	<6%
Hypopyon	0.3% (3/806)	<1.8%
Endophthalmitis	0.1% (1/806)	<1%
Posterior dislocation of the IOL	0.1% (1/806)	<1%
Pupil block	0.1% (1/806)	<1%
Retinal detachment	1.2% (10/806)	<1.8%
Secondary surgical intervention	0.3% (3/806)	<2.6%
Persistent		
Corneal edema	0.2% (2/806)	<0.8%
Cystoid macular edema	0	<2.2%
Iritis	0.1% (1/806) (Preop Iridocyclitis)	<1.8%
Raised intraocular pressure resistant to therapy	0	<1.8%

below (Fig. 6.5). The occurrence of adverse effects after implantation of the "bag-in-the-lens" lens is shown in Table 6.1 (Fig. 6.6).

In this large cohort, we found no opacification of the visual axis in adults. The edge of the capsule escaped from the groove of the implant in four children (we did not yet know about the possible issue of a smaller Berger space in children), but in all other cases, the axis also remained clear. The absence of proliferation of cells on the visual axis validated our previous studies: closing off the capsular bag-in-the-lens groove and constraining the proliferation outside the visual axis. This has also been shown by postmortem analysis of the capsular bag after implantation of BIL (Fig. 6.6).

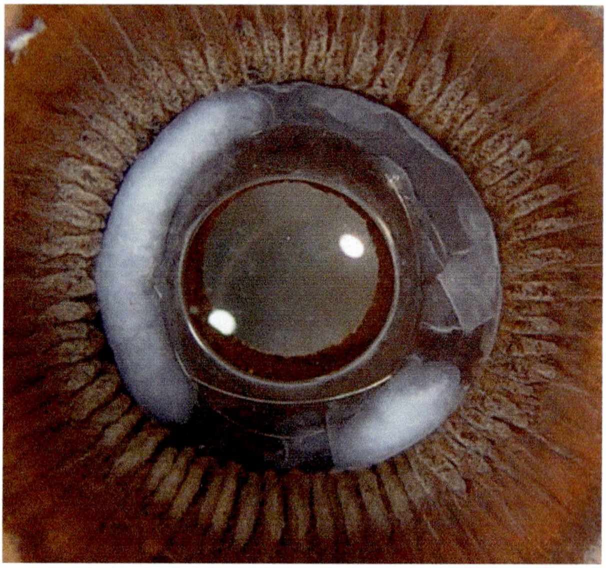

Fig. 6.6 Photo of a dissected postmortem eye, death occurred 2 years after implantation of BIL (view of the posterior chamber while looking toward the anterior chamber) [38]

A priori, the cohort was too small and the follow-up too short for the accurate determination of the retinal detachment (RD) rate after implantation and comparison with that of the literature [26–29]. The ISO standard establishes a maximum safety rate of 1.8% for 300 eyes at 1 year. We enlarged the patient cohort to allow for the proper evaluation of RD after bag-in-the-lens IOL implantation in 1323 eyes with an average follow-up of 44.75 months (range 0–152 months). RD was found in 19 eyes (1.44%). The 1-year RD incidence was 0.49% (5 RD cases in 1024 eyes) (0.00% in patients without risk factors). The 2-year cumulative RD incidence was 0.84% (9 RD cases in 931 eyes; 0.15% without risk factors). Four clinically significant risk factors were confirmed: male gender, young age at time of surgery (<60 years), axial myopia (axial length ≥25 mm), and history of contralateral RD in the total cohort.

6.6 Visual Performance

In our cohort of 295 eyes, 195 patients were followed for more than 1 year (mean 33.1 ± 14.7 months (12–84 months)). Postoperative visual acuity was 0.94 ± 0.18 decimal Snellen, and the histogram of the distribution is shown in Fig. 6.7. In 91.5%

of the patients, the visual acuity was better than 0.8. The postoperative refraction was −0.19 ± 0.84 D (−3.5 to +5 D) for the sphere and −0.58 ± 0.77 D for the cylinder (Fig. 6.8). The spherical equivalent was −0.48 ± 0.82 D for a target refraction of −0.24 ± 0.71 D. The A constant was adjusted from a value of 119.0 for the 169 patients to 118.4 for the next 459 and finally 118.2 for all of the others. Finally, an A constant of 118.0 to 118.2 was the best fit.

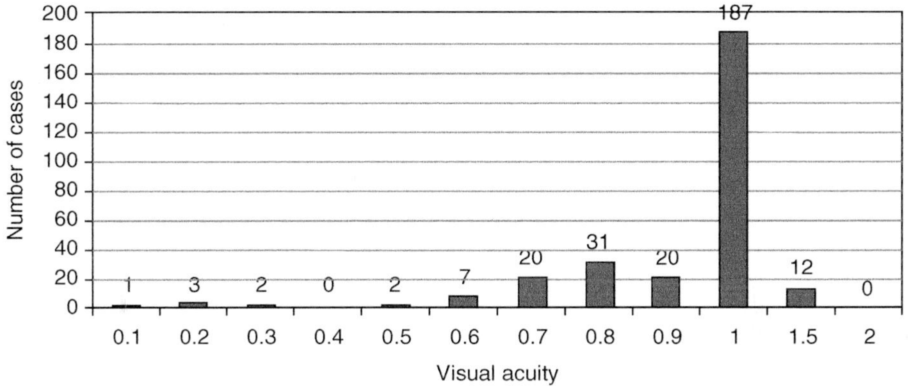

Fig. 6.7 Histogram of postoperative visual acuity

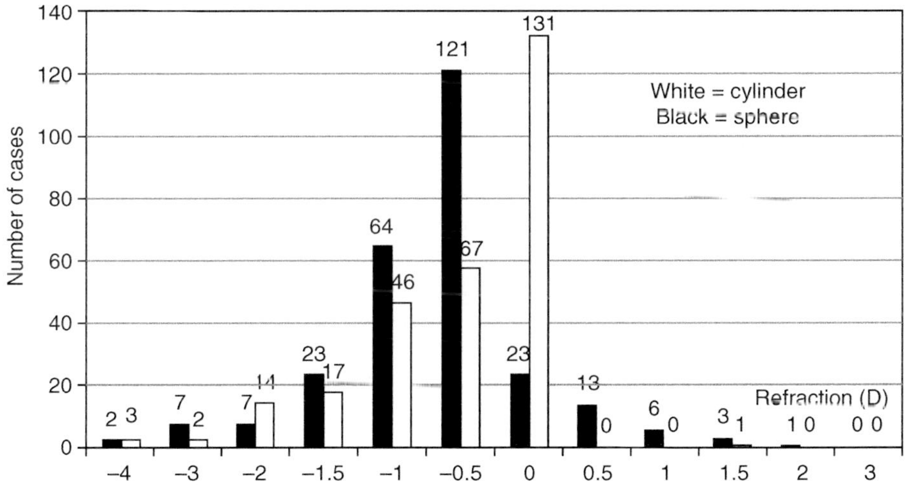

Fig. 6.8 Distribution of spherical and cylindrical powers after implantation of BIL

6.7 Measurement of Lens Centration

The measurement of the BIL centration was made using a utility developed by J. Rozema [30]. The center of the lens is determined by an elliptical fit of the edge of the implant. The determination of the pupil and limbic center is made by the same type of adjustment. We found a mean center (centroid of optical centers) 0.3040.17 mm at −24.9113°, that is to say voluntarily inferonasal for the conservation of the angle kappa. The distribution of the optical centers is contained below the threshold determined as inducing a decrease in visual acuity: 0.7 mm [31].

6.8 Measurement of Lens Tilt

The tilt measurement was made by a Scheimpflug imaging method (Pentacam, Oculus, Germany). The image was calibrated using the groove pixel diameter (5 mm) to calibrate the pixel size. The procedure for determining the tilt of the lens was to find the axis in which the lens was flatter and the axis in which the lens was steeper (Fig. 6.9). We were able to determine the tilt of the implant by using the inverse cosine ratio of the distance between the highest part of the groove to the optical axis (in the most inclined configuration) and the radius of the implant.

This method applied to 30 eyes implanted with BIL allowed us to determine a tilt of 7.2 ± 2.9°, from 3° to 13°. The inclination with respect to the horizontal plane of the cut in which the implant was more inclined was, on average, 4.83 ± 34.9° temporally (Fig. 6.10).

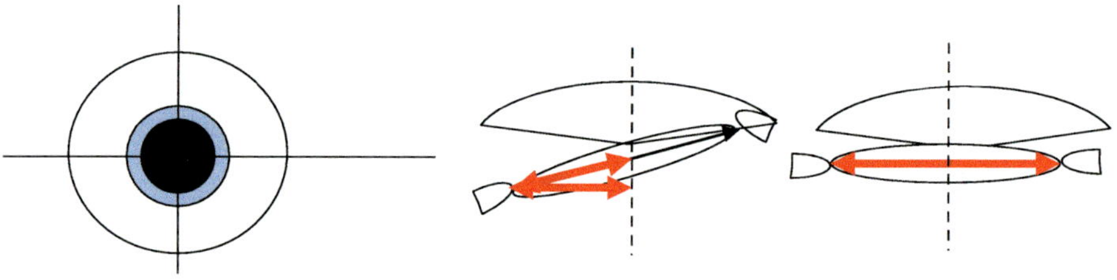

Fig. 6.9 Method of calculating the tilt in the eye

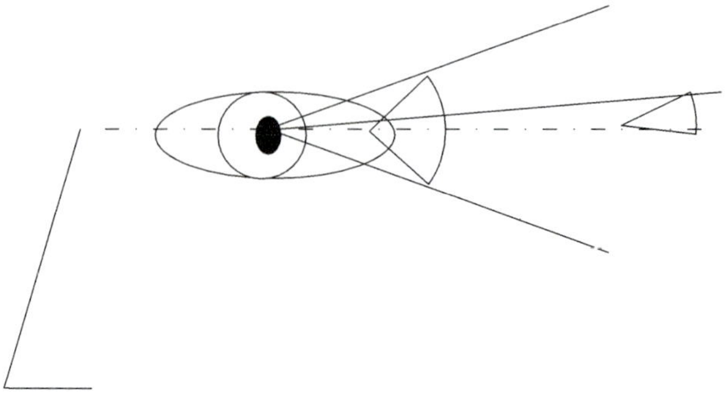

Fig. 6.10 The maximum physiological tilt has always been found between −35° and 35°, with an average of 5° in the coronal section

The Scheimpflug imaging method does not dissociate the rotation of the eyeball from the tilt, and we never observed tilt in the vertical section. This is why we qualified this method biased. In the horizontal position, the natural tilt in both phakic and pseudophakic patients is temporal for the right eye as for the left eye. This is reflected in the MRI images (Fig. 6.11b) and has also been proposed in the literature [32]. We therefore could not measure the tilt of this implant adequately. However, we have been able to highlight that the use of Scheimpflug for measuring the tilt of the implant in the eye was inappropriate because this technique also measures the natural tilt. The only reliable method for measuring tilt is Purkinje's reflections [33, 34], which look for reflections on different surfaces of the eye, but this method is not commercially available (Fig. 6.12).

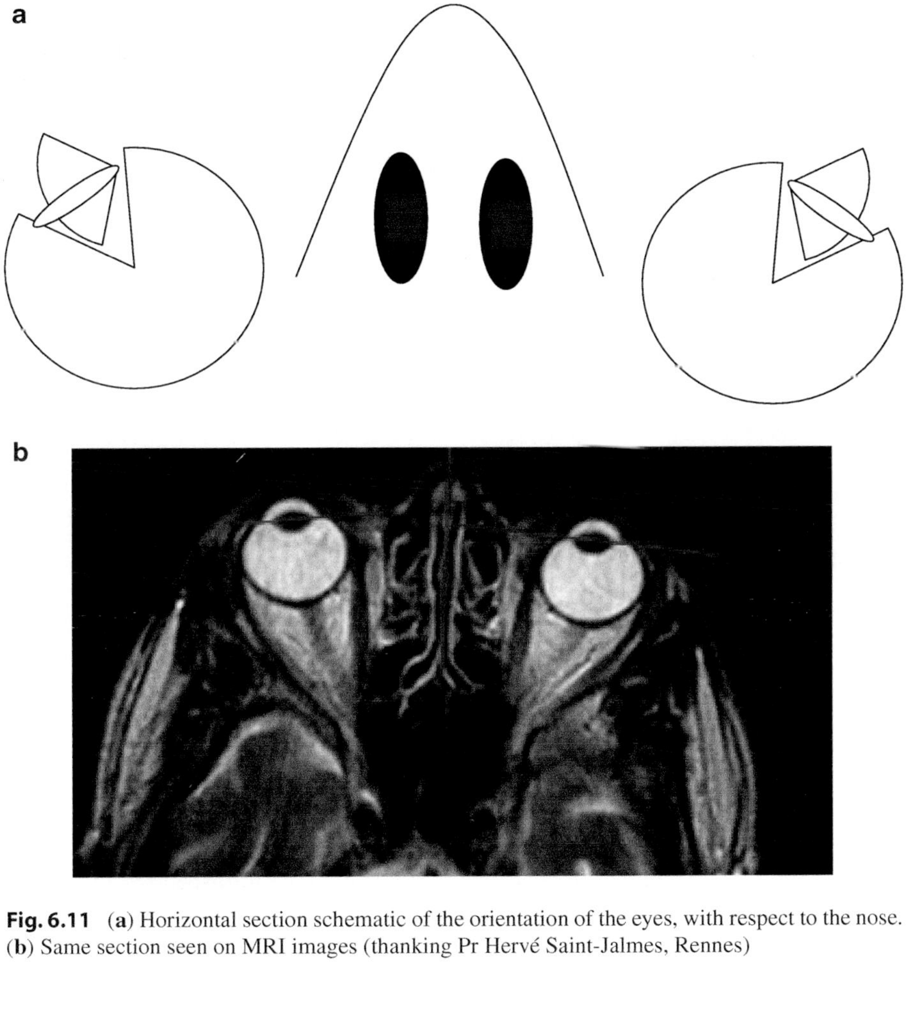

Fig. 6.11 (**a**) Horizontal section schematic of the orientation of the eyes, with respect to the nose. (**b**) Same section seen on MRI images (thanking Pr Hervé Saint-Jalmes, Rennes)

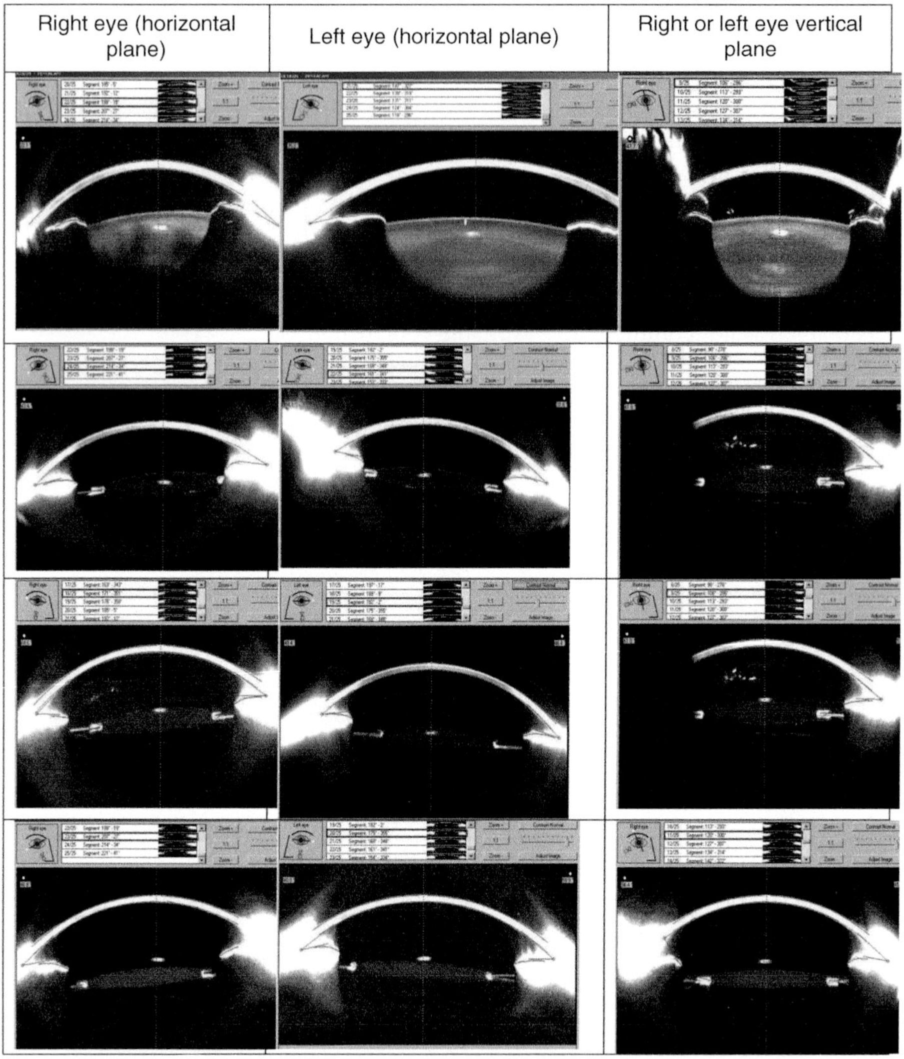

Fig. 6.12 Scheimpflug images of the anterior chamber of the eye: we see the temporal inclination of the implant always in the same cut (5° to the horizontal) while the tilt is absent in the vertical sections

6.9 Rotational Stability of the Lens

Our rotational study included 59 eyes of 49 patients with a mean age of 68.0 ± 11.9 years. The rotation over time was made by the retrospective analysis of photos, calibrated with the optical diameter and the optical center. The edge of the haptic was marked by triangulation with respect to a fixed anatomical landmark. The rotation was almost nil between 1 day (0.052.02°) and 5 weeks and 0.361.39°

between 5 weeks and 6 months. No correlation was found between implant power and rotation ($P = 0.862$, t test) [35].

6.10 Developing the Toric BIL Implant

The design of a toric implant in 2005 also required the creation of a new calculator. The details of this calculator are covered in a separate chapter. The theory is covered here. The residual astigmatism due to the inaccuracy of orientation of the axis of the toroid implant cylinder is defined by:

$$\text{Cyl} = 2\Delta K \cos\left(\theta_{\text{k}} - \theta_{\text{IOL}}\right) \tag{6.1}$$

The direction of the power axis of residual astigmatism is defined by the following:

$$\theta_{\text{Cyl}} = \frac{\theta_{\text{k}} + \theta_{\text{IOL}}}{2} \tag{6.2}$$

Equations 6.1 and 6.2 determine the residual astigmatism (power and direction) in the event of misalignment of the implant on the corneal axis. The alignment error in diopters can be expressed as a function of the misalignment ($\theta_{\text{k}} - \theta_{\text{IOL}}$).

$$\text{Alignment error} = 2\cos\left(\theta_{\text{k}} - \theta_{\text{IOL}}\right) \tag{6.3}$$

This function is drawn and shown in Fig. 6.13. Here we are referring to the power axis, that is to say at 90° of the axes indicated on the implant. An error of ±5° in the alignment of the implant thus induces an error of −20% on the correction of astigmatism. More generally, on the basis of this curve, we were able to determine the

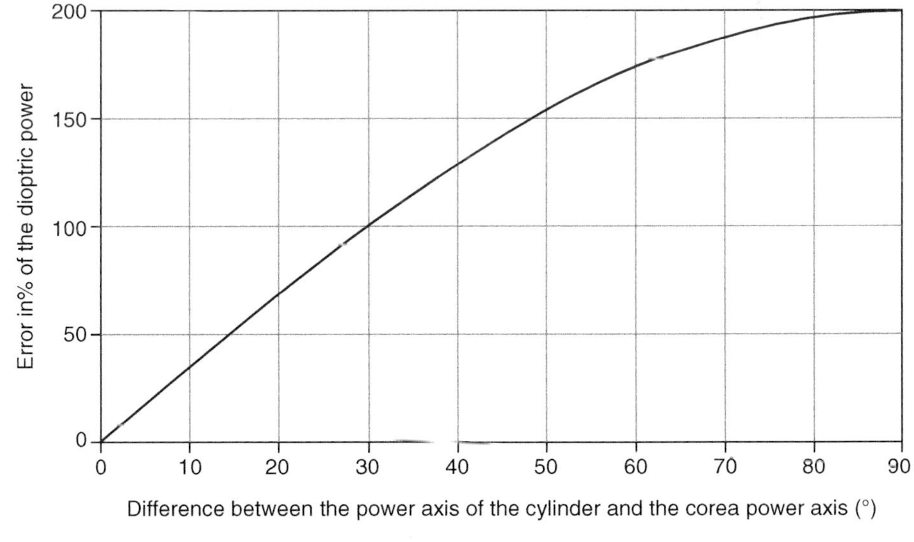

Fig. 6.13 Percentage of the error in % of the dioptric power of the implant as a function of the misalignment in degrees (°) between the power axis of the cornea and the implant

extent to which the intraocular correction of irregular astigmatism brought a benefit to the patient. In short, if the lens rotated beyond 10° in irregular astigmatism, the theoretical error is close to 40% and will result in almost half of the uncorrected astigmatism. The question to ask in these cases is: is there a real benefit to intraocular correction by inducing non-corrective HOAs?

We examined 53 eyes of the first 29 patients implanted consecutively [36]. The average follow-up was 5.14 ± 5.36 months (thus greater than the healing time of the cornea). Cylindrical correction ranged from 1 D to 8 D with an average astigmatic correction of 2.96 D. Preoperative visual acuity was 0.58 ± 0.25. The postoperative visual acuity with correction is on average 0.85 ± 0.21 ($p < 0.05$). Postoperative visual acuity, although satisfactory, remained limited in certain cases. It was with these cases that we developed a methodology for predicting the postoperative situation by using Holladay's "Holladay Diagnosis Summary" [37] method to detect irregular astigmatism. 82% of the astigmatisms have been corrected. The average postoperative sphere was 0.33 ± 0.87 D, that is, slightly hypermetropic. This led us to generate more precise calculations for the spherocylindrical implant. The analysis of the quality of the toric correction was made according to the method of Alpins and is shown below (Table 6.2). It is the toric conformation that really takes advantage of the BIL design because if the alignment of the implant is ever lost, it can be adjusted postoperatively no matter how long it has been since the primary surgery. The lens can be easily rotated back to its correct axis, even after Elschnig pearl formation.

Table 6.2 Analysis of astigmatism using the method of Alpins

Parameter	
Targeted astigmatism (D)	
Amplitude (mean ± standard deviation)	3,20 ± 1,36
Mean vector (standard @ axis)	3,20 D@ −2,45°
Surgically induced astigmatism (SIA)	
Amplitude (mean ± standard deviation)	3,26 ± 1,51 D
Mean vector (standard @ axis)	3,26 D@ −2,16°
Vector difference	
Amplitude (mean ± standard deviation)	0,56 ± 0,79 D
Mean vector (standard @ axis)	0,56 D@ 4,38°
Amplitude of the error	0,05 ± 0,49 D
Direction of error	0,26 ± 0,89°
Correction index	1,01 ± 0,15
Index of success	0,18 ± 0,26
Percentage of corrected astigmatism	101%
Percentage of successfully corrected astigmatism	82%

6.11 Conclusion

Our clinical studies confirm the in vivo and in vitro results showing that the "Bag-in-the-Lens" intraocular lens is a valid option to eradicate PCO, provided that the surgery is performed properly. The tight fit of the two capsules into the peripheral groove of the IOL blocks the migration of the lens epithelial cells and their proliferation is confined to the remaining peripheral capsular bag. The visual axis remains transparent in all eyes, including those of children. We have also shown that the implant could be centered correctly and that it did not rotate in the eye. Incorporating an astigmatic correction into the optics of this very stable implant in the eye was the next step.

Overall, designing and implementing the lens has been an iterative process, but our results show that it has been worthwhile, as the lens confers excellent results, not only in PCO prevention but also in centration and rotation in both children and adults.

References

1. Nishi O. Incidence of posterior capsule opacification in eyes with and without posterior chamber intraocular lenses. J Cataract Refract Surg. 1986;12:519–22.
2. Apple DJ. Harold Ridley, MA, MD, FRCS; a golden anniversary celebration and a golden age (editorial). Arch Ophthalmol. 1999;117:827–8.
3. Pandey SK, Apple DJ, Werner L, et al. Posterior capsule opacification: a review of the aetiopathogenesis, experimental and clinical studies and factors for prevention. Indian J. 2005;16:2–7.
4. Apple DJ, Solomon KD, Tetz MR, et al. Posterior capsule opacification. Surv Ophthalmol. 1992;37:73–116.
5. Rakic JM, Galand A, Vrensen GFJM. Separation of fibers from the capsule enhances mitotic activity of human lens epithelium. Exp Eye Res. 1997;64:67–72.
6. Meacock WR, Spalton DJ, Boyce J, Marshall J. The effect of posterior capsule opacification on visual function. Invest Ophthalmol Vis Sci. 2003;44:4665–9.
7. Aslam TM, Aspinall P, Dhillon B. Posterior capsule morphology determinants of visual function. Graefes Arch Clin Exp Ophthalmol. 2003;241:208–12.
8. Aslam TM, Devlin H, Dhillon B. Use of Nd :YAG laser capsulotomy. Surv Ophthalmol. 2003;48:594–612.
9. Billotte C, Berdeaux G. Adverse clinical consequences of neodymium: YAG laser treatment of posterior capsule opacification. J Cataract Refract Surg. 2004;30:2064–71.
10. De Groot V, Vrensen G, Willekens B, Van Tenten Y, Tassignon MJ. In vitro study on the closure of posterior Capsulorhexis in the human eye. Investig Ophthalmol Vis Sci. 2003;44:2076–83.
11. Abhilakh Missier KA, Nuijts RMMA, Tjia KF. Posterior capsule opacification: silicone plate-haptic versus Acrysof intraocular lenses. J Cataract Refract Surg. 2003;29:1569–74.
12. Hollick EJ, Spalton DJ, Ursell PG, et al. The effect of polymethylmethacrylate, silicone, and polyacrylic intraocular lenses on posterior capsular opacification 3 years after cataract surgery. Ophthalmology. 1999;106:49 54. discussion by RC Drews, 54 55.
13. Sundelin K, Friberg-Riad Y, Östberg A, Sjöstrand J. Posterior capsule opacification with Acrysof and poly(methylmethacrylate) intraocular lenses. Comparative study with a 3-year follow-up. J Cataract Refract Surg. 2001;27:1586–90.
14. Ernest PH. Posterior capsule opacification and neodymium:YAG capsulotomy rates with AcrySof acrylic and PhacoFlex II silicone intraocular lenses. J Cataract Refract Surg. 2003;29:1546–50.
15. Gimbel HV, Neuhann T. Developments, advantages and methods of the continuous circular capsulorhexis technique. J Cataract Refract Surg. 1990;16:31–7.

16. Spalton DJ. Posterior capsular opacification after cataract surgery. Eye. 1999;13:489–92.
17. Dana MR, Chatzistefanou K, Schaumberg DA, et al. Posterior capsule opacification after cataract surgery in patients with uveitis. Ophthalmology. 1997;104:1387–93.
18. United States Patent 6, 027, 531 (Tassignon – February 22, 2000): Intraocular lens and method for preventing secondary opacification.
19. Tassignon MJ, De Groot V, Vrensen G. Bag-in-the-lens implantation of intra-ocular lenses. J Cataract Refract Surg. 2002;28:1182–288.
20. De Groot V, Tassignon J, Vrensen GFJM. Effect of bag-in-the-lens implantation on posterior capsule opacification in human donor eyes and rabbit eyes. J Cataract Refract Surg. 2005;31:398–405.
21. De Groot V, Leysen I, Neuhann T, Gobin L, Tassignon MJ. One year follow-up of the "bag-in-the-lens" implantation in 60 eyes. J Cataract Refract Surg. 2006.; In Press.
22. Tassignon MJ, Rozema JJ, Gobin L. Ring-shaped caliper for better anterior capsulorhexis sizing and centration. J Cataract Refract Surg. 2006;32(8):1253–5.
23. Leysen I, Coeckelbergh T, Gobin L, et al. Cumulative Nd:YAG laser rate after bag-in-the-lens implantation compared to lens-in-the-bag implantation. J Cataract Refract Surg. 2006.; In Press.
24. Leysen I, Coeckelbergh T, Gobin L, Smet H, Daniel Y, De Groot V, Tassignon MJ. Cumulative neodymium:YAG laser rates after bag-in-the-lens and lens-in-the-bag intraocular lens implantation: comparative study. J Cataract Refract Surg. 2006;32(12):2085–90.
25. Tassignon MJ, Gobin L, Mathysen D, Van Looveren J, De Groot V. Clinical outcomes of cataract surgery after bag-in-the-lens intraocular lens implantation following ISO standard 11979-7:2006. J Cataract Refract Surg. 2011;37(12):2120–9.
26. Lois N, Wong D. Pseudophakic retinal detachment, major review. Surv Ophthalmol. 2003;48(5):467–87.
27. Bhagwandien AC, Cheng YY, Wolfs RC, van Meurs JC, Luyten GP. Relationship between retinal detachment and biometry in 4262 cataractous eyes. Ophthalmology. 2006;113(4):643–9.
28. Tielsch JM, Legro MW, Cassard SD, Schein OD, Javitt JC, Singer AE, Bass EB, Steinberg EP. Risk factors for retinal detachment after cataract surgery. A population-based case-control study. Ophthalmology. 1996;103(10):1537–45.
29. Tuft SJ, Minassian D, Sullivan P. Risk factors for retinal detachment after cataract surgery: a case-control study. Ophthalmology. 2006;113(4):650–6.
30. Verbruggen KH, Rozema JJ, Gobin L, Coeckelbergh T, De Groot V, Tassignon MJ. Intraocular lens centration and visual outcomes after bag-in-the-lens implantation. J Cataract Refract Surg. 2007;33(7):1267–72.
31. Hayashi K, Hayashi H, Nakao F, Hayashi F. Correlation between pupillary size and intraocular lens decentration and visual acuity of a zonal-progressive multifocal lens and a monofocal lens. Ophthalmology. 2001;108(11):2011–7.
32. Cheng HM, Singh OS, et al. Shape of the myopic eye with high resolution MRI. Optom Vis Sci. 1992;69:698–701.
33. de Castro A, Rosales P, Marcos S. Tilt and decentration of intraocular lenses in vivo from Purkinje and Scheimpflug imaging. Validation study. J Cataract Refract Surg. 2007;33(3):418–29.
34. Marcos S, Rosales P, Llorente L, Jiménez-Alfaro I. Change in corneal aberrations after cataract surgery with 2 types of aspherical intraocular lenses. J Cataract Refract Surg. 2007;33(2):217–26.
35. Rozema JJ, Gobin L, Verbruggen K, Tassignon MJ. Changes in rotation after implantation of a bag-in-the-lens intraocular lens. J Cataract Refract Surg. 2009;35(8):1385–8.
36. Tassignon MJ, Gobin L, Mathysen D, Van Looveren J. Clinical results after spherotoric intraocular lens implantation using the bag-in-the-lens technique. J Cataract Refract Surg. 2011;37(5):830–4.
37. Holladay JT. Corneal topography using the Holladay Diagnostic Summary. J Cataract Refract Surg. 1997;23(2):209–21.
38. Werner L, Tassignon MJ, Gobin L, Rozema J, Davis D, Brubaker J. Bag-in-the-lens: first pathological analysis of a human eye obtained postmortem. J Cataract Refract Surg. 2008;34(12):2163–5.

The Evolution of the Anterior Capsulotomy

7

Richard Packard

7.1 Introduction

In 1747, the world of cataract surgery was changed by Jacques Daviel when instead of pushing the cataractous lens backwards into the vitreous, he extracted the opaque nucleus from the eye. In order to do this, he had to open the lens capsule which he did by tearing it crudely with a cystitome. Over the course of the following two centuries and more, the techniques to open the capsule hardly changed. The invention of the intraocular lens changed things. Harold Ridley, who first placed his disc intraocular lens (IOL) in the posterior chamber, had no idea if this lens was inside or outside of the capsular bag. The lens was inherently unstable partly because of this but also due to its excessive weight when compared with a modern IOL.

Cornelius Binkhorst, one of the most important pioneers of implantology, was the first to realise that if you could fixate the IOL into the capsular bag, then it would be more stable and less likely to irritate ocular tissues. Accordingly, he designed an IOL which he called iridocapsular to be partly supported by the iris but mainly by the capsular bag. Binkhorst's problem was that he could not decide on the best shape for the capsular opening (Fig. 7.1).

Others tried to produce different ways to open the capsule, such as Albert Galand's envelope technique. Here a linear opening was made proximal to the incision and after the removal of the lens nucleus, cortical clearance and IOL insertion, the anterior capsule was torn open in a continuous manner after making a small scissor cut at the capsular edge (Fig. 7.2).

R. Packard (✉)
Arnott Eye Associates, London, UK
e-mail: mail@eyequack.vossnet.co.uk

M.-J. Tassignon et al. (eds.), *Innovative Implantation Technique*,
https://doi.org/10.1007/978-3-030-03086-5_7

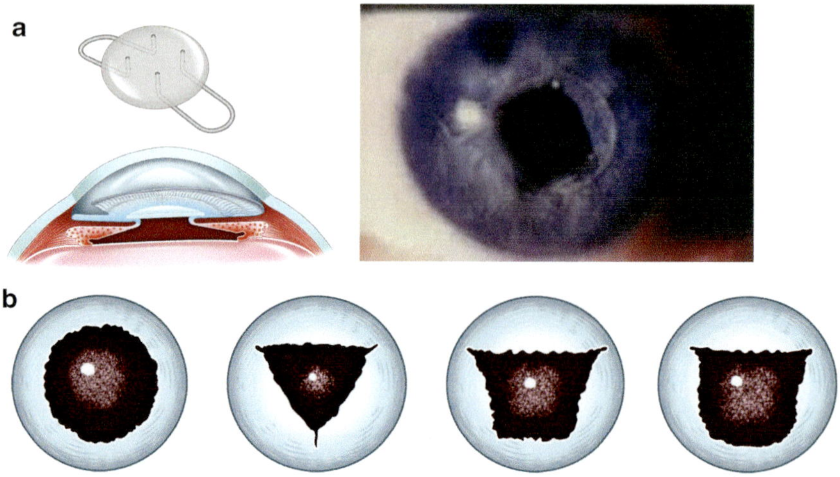

Fig. 7.1 Binkhorst iridocapsular lens and capsulotomy shapes

Fig. 7.2 Galand envelope capsulotomy

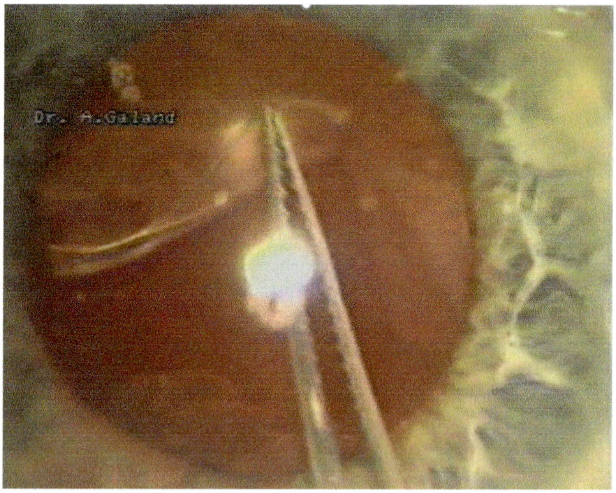

7.2 Early Approaches to the Capsulorhexis

At the beginning of the 1970s, the inventor of phacoemulsification, Charles Kelman, used a different method to gain access to the lens nucleus to emulsify it intracamerally through a small incision. He tore the capsule in a triangular manner, the so-called "Christmas tree" capsulotomy (Fig. 7.3) and then trimmed the third side of the triangle with scissors.

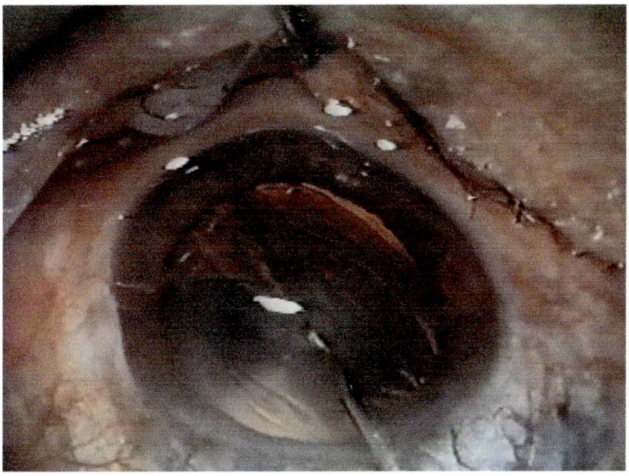

Fig. 7.3 Christmas tree capsulotomy

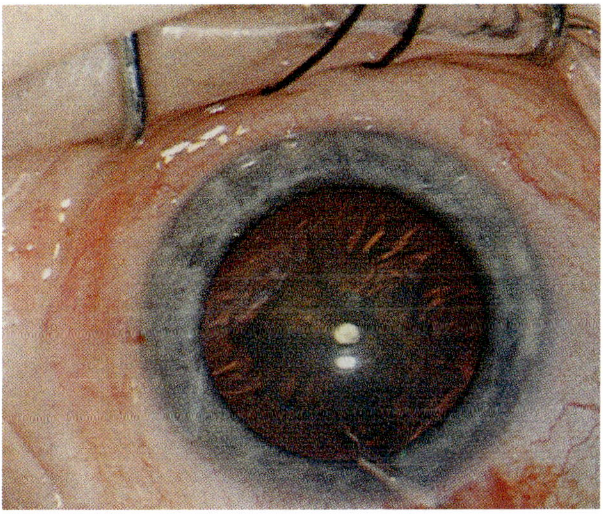

Fig. 7.4 Can opener capsulotomy

When in the late 1970s Richard Kratz wanted to perform iris plane phacoemulsification and tilt the lens nucleus, he devised a round capsulotomy with a serrated edge called the "can opener" (Fig. 7.4). It was also felt that this type of capsulotomy would hold a posterior chamber IOL better.

However, none of these methods (and other attempts to create a capsular opening) was immune from tearing at the edge. The surgeon, when implanting an IOL, could also not be certain that the whole of the IOL was in the bag or that it would stay there as the capsule contracted in the weeks and months following cataract surgery.

The first attempt to use a different modality was made in the early 1980s by the inventor of the YAG laser for posterior capsulotomy, Danielle Aron Rosa, using her laser to open the anterior capsule. Multiple punctures were made in a circular pattern. Unfortunately, unless the cataract surgery was carried out immediately, the intraocular pressure would build as the soft lens matter expanded due to hydration by aqueous and surgery, therefore, became difficult. This method was quickly abandoned.

7.3 The Continuous Curvilinear Capsulorhexis

The solution to remedy these problems turned out to be a continuous circular tear in the capsule. For most ophthalmologists, two surgeons have been credited with pioneering the technique called continuous curvilinear capsulorhexis (CCC); the story is more complex than that however. Thomas Neuhann in Germany and Howard Gimbel in Canada have received the most recognition for this and certainly produced the first paper to appear in the peer reviewed literature [1]. However, across the world and at the same time Kimiya Shimizu was doing something very similar. Each of these three surgeons added a part of the name for this capsulotomy. Gimbel called it continuous, Shimizu added the word curvilinear, and Neuhann coined the term capsulorhexis. Although these surgeons had similar ideas, their approaches to the creation of the CCC and the instruments they used differed.

Charles Kelman had designed an instrument called the irrigating cystitome and this is what Howard Gimbel had used. He modified the can opener technique by pulling on the capsule to create the tear, but did not allow the edge to become serrated, instead it remained continuous (Fig. 7.5). He performed this under viscoelastic.

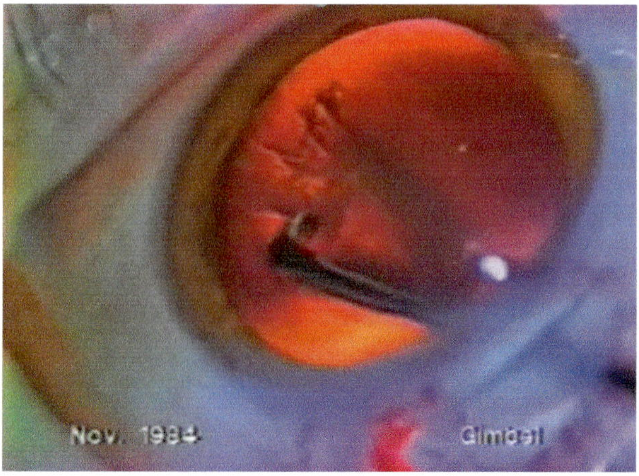

Fig. 7.5 Gimbel capsulotomy

Kimiya Shimizu used a bent 30-gauge needle under viscoelastic to create a tear and then a flap of anterior capsule. He then folded this flap onto the untorn capsule and directed the tear in a curvilinear manner with the tip of the needle, very similarly to how many surgeons do it today (Fig. 7.6).

This author first observed the technique that Thomas Neuhann first used for his capsulorhexis at a conference in Bordeaux in 1986. It was performed during live surgery by another German surgeon, Jurgen Greite. He had been taught by Thomas Neuhann as they both worked in Munich. The Neuhann technique was performed with irrigation initially with a straight 26-gauge needle. This needle created a small T-shaped opening in the anterior capsule just in front of the main incision site. Then a curved needle with a bent tip was inserted into the eye, and the small flaps created by the capsular incision were stroked up each side to create the CCC (Fig. 7.7).

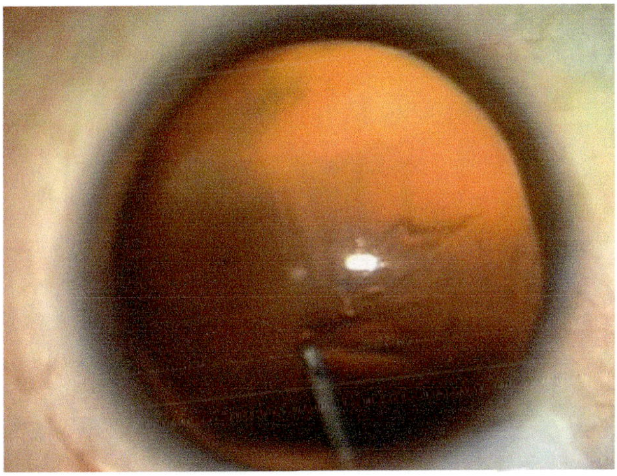

Fig. 7.6 Shimizu capsulotomy

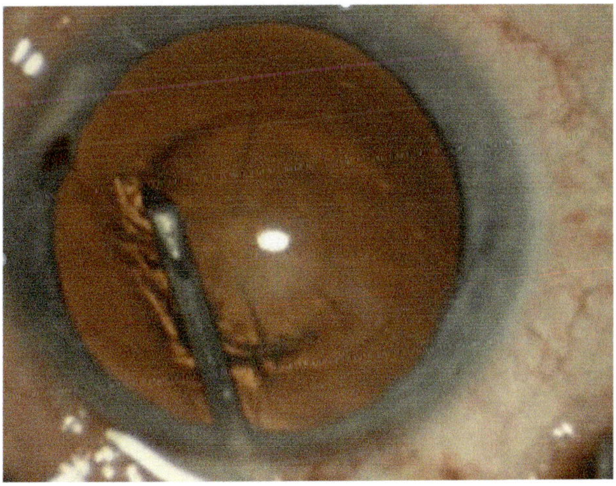

Fig. 7.7 Neuhann capsulotomy

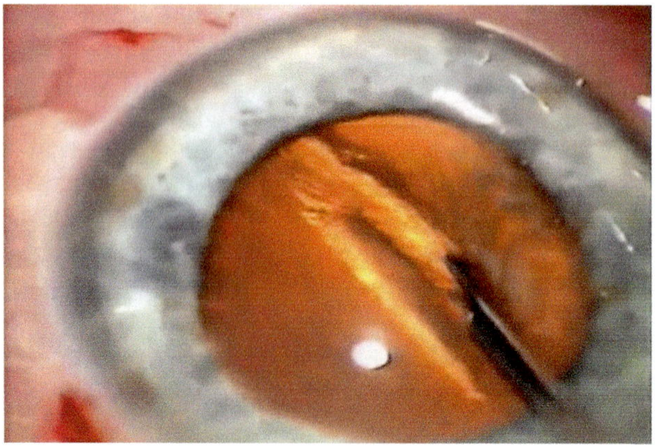

Fig. 7.8 Fercho capsulotomy

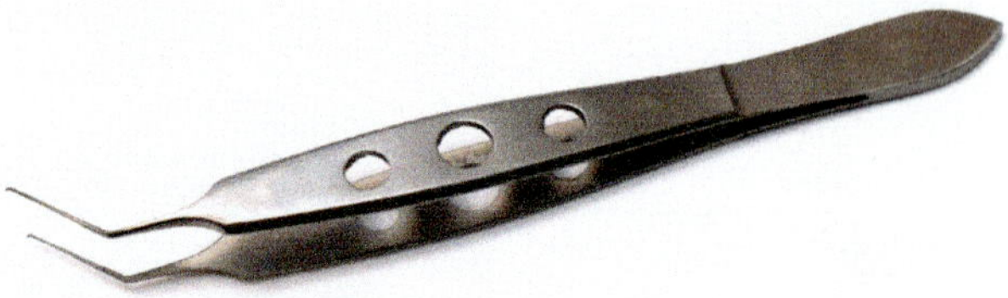

Fig. 7.9 Utrata forceps

But were these three really the first to perform a CCC? It does not seem so. A surgeon in the United States named Calvin Fercho was almost certainly the first to do this. He started using a continuous tear in the late 1970s, and this was documented by a number of surgeons who watched him operate [2]. He did not present on this though, due to his having to take time out for ill health until 1986. His technique was a sort of combination of that used by Gimbel and Shimizu. He used an irrigating cystitome with the irrigation initially, later on under viscoelastic, and tore the capsule with this and then directed the flap to make the CCC (Fig. 7.8).

Although many surgeons still use only a needle or cystitome to create the CCC, many use forceps. The first forceps specifically designed to perform this capsulotomy were designed by Peter Utrata and appeared in 1988. Although there have been many variations on this theme, the basic design is still used widely today (Fig. 7.9). The reason that many surgeons prefer to use forceps is the greater controllability they afford to the surgeon.

One of the unintended consequences of adopting the CCC was in the way that the nucleus was removed from the eye with phacoemulsification. Tilting up the nucleus, as in the Kratz technique, was now much more difficult and so new methods were needed. This led to "chip and flip", "divide and conquer", "phaco chop", "phaco pre-chop" and many others. The major advantages proffered were that the edge of the capsulotomy was much stronger and had less of a tendency to tear out. Irrigation aspiration was safer, given that there were no torn edges to suck into the aspiration port. The IOL could now be reliably placed within the capsular bag and was likely to stay there well-centred.

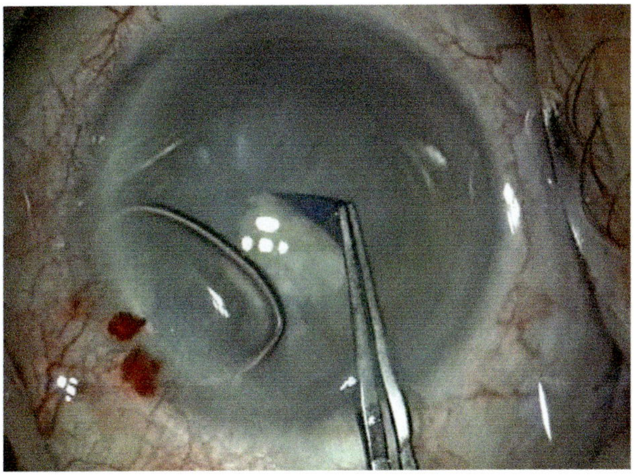

Fig. 7.10 Capsulotomy with trypan blue stained capsule

This new capsulotomy needed a good red reflex to be easy enough to perform, and certainly a hypermature white cataract presented a major challenge to even the most experienced surgeon. Many would revert to a "can opener" capsular opening in these cases. A device using high-frequency radio diathermy was invented by Kloti to overcome this problem. It made the capsulotomy in white cataracts much easier, but the capsular edge was not as strong as a CCC. The problem of how to deal with these mature lenses with a poor red reflex was solved by using a vital stain trypan blue to stain the anterior capsule. Although Gerrit Melles is generally credited with this idea, Minas Coroneo first used this while working in the Australian outback operating on aboriginal patients. He holds a patent on the idea (Fig. 7.10).

7.4 Advances in the Capsulotomy Techniques

Although getting a complete CCC is relatively straightforward for the experienced surgeon, are there ways to make the size and circularity of the capsular opening more precise? A number of ways have been described to do this. Marie Jose Tassignon has designed a ring that is slipped into the eye and centred on the pupil to act as a guide for the surgeon (Fig. 7.11). Alternatively, there is the Verus capsulotomy guide; this is a soft flat circular device which is placed on the anterior capsule and acts as a guide for the tearing of the capsule (Fig. 7.12). Marking the cornea with specially sized circular instrument can also aid the surgeon (Fig. 7.13).

Heads-up displays in the surgeon's view down an operating microscope of a circle displayed on the cornea, as provided in devices like Verion (Alcon, USA) or Callisto (Zeiss, Germany), can also help to achieve greater accuracy (Fig. 7.14). A recent paper by Haeussler-Sinangin et al. has shown that even with experienced surgeons, these devices can improve the CCC [2]:

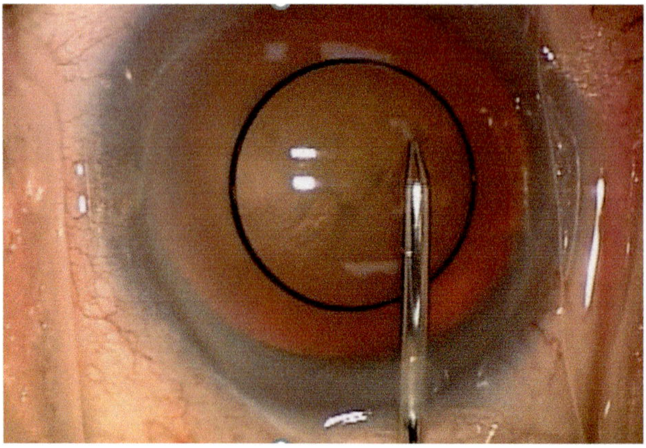

Fig. 7.11 Tassignon capsulotomy ring

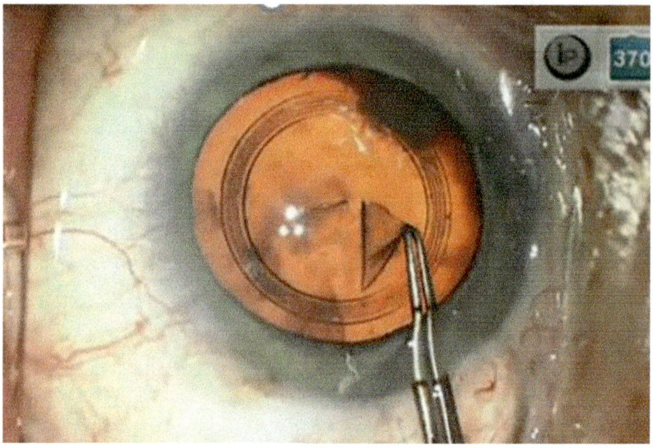

Fig. 7.12 Verus capsulotomy ring

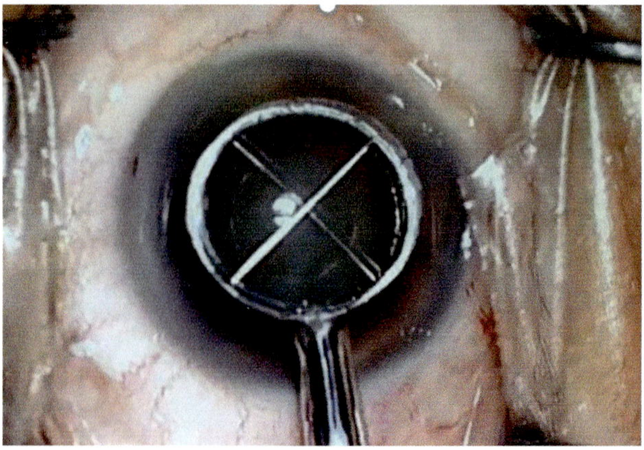

Fig. 7.13 Corneal ring marker

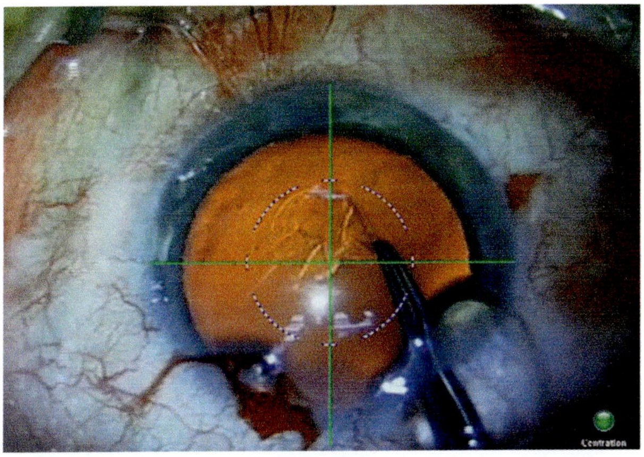

Fig. 7.14 Digital overlay in miroscope view

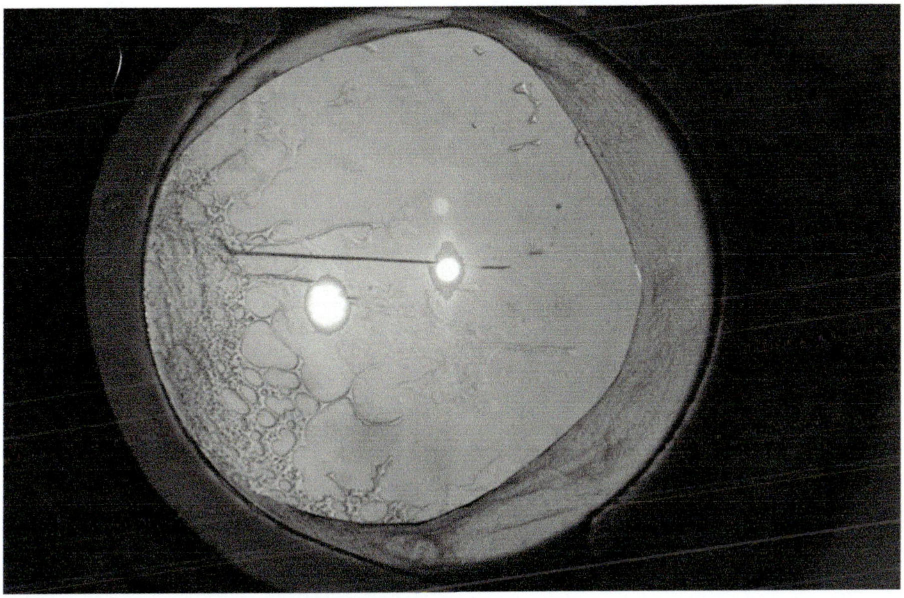

Fig. 7.15 Asymmetric capsulotomy with PCO

- IOL centration and stability particularly for multifocal and toric IOLs
- IOL effective lens position
- Overlapping of the IOL edge with the capsule
- Shrink wrapping of the IOL by the capsule to lessen PCO

Emma Hollick with David Spalton's team has shown that a poorly centred CCC, without good edge coverage of the IOL, leads to earlier posterior capsular opacification (Fig. 7.15) [3]. Little changed for another decade until the initial use of the femtosecond laser for cataract surgery in 2008 by Zoltan Nagy in Hungary

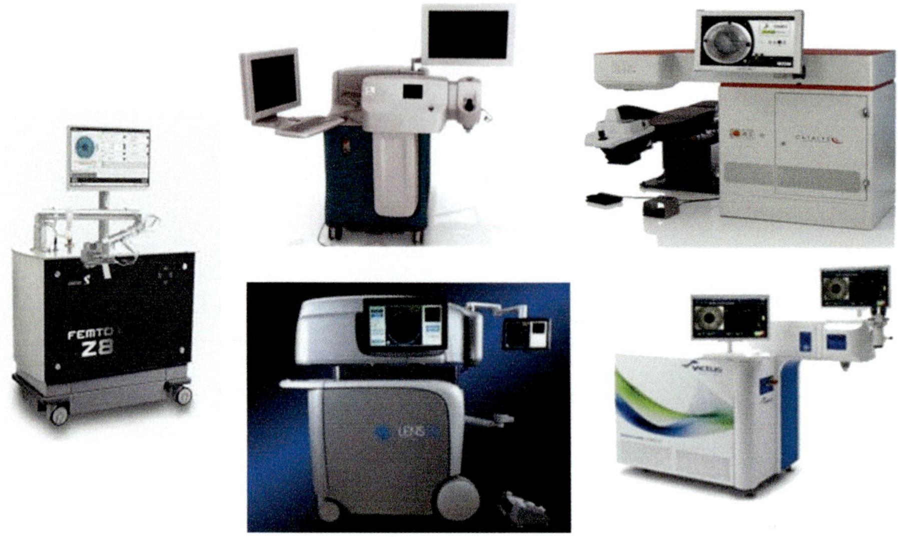

Fig. 7.16 Femtosecond lasers

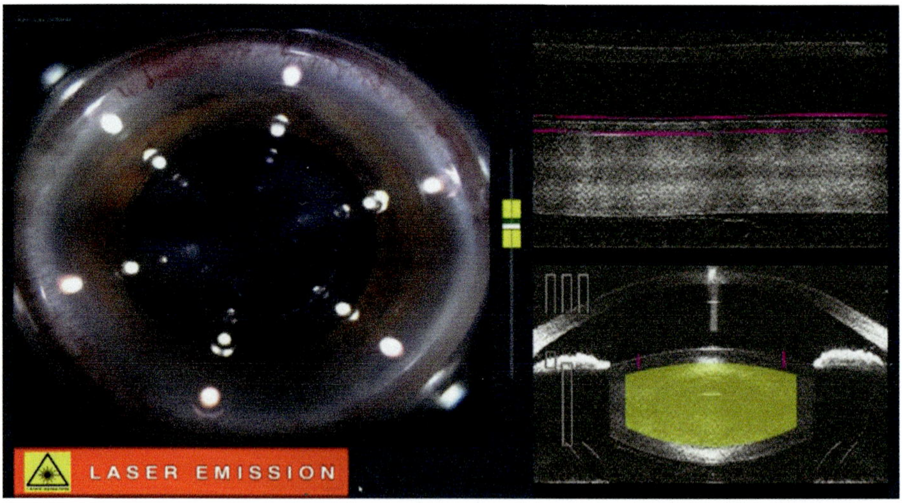

Fig. 7.17 Imaging during capsulotomy with femtosecond laser

(Fig. 7.16). This was a fundamental change in the way that the anterior capsulotomy was performed. For the first time, we could make capsulotomies of a given size which were truly circular, in a given position, with little risk of tear-out during the capsulotomy, without the variables of a manual technique. The imaging devices built into the machine assist in all of this (Fig. 7.17).

However, there were caveats with this new technology. A second room might be needed for the laser, something which interfered with the surgical flow. Both the cost of the device and the running costs are high and there is a click fee for patients. To date, no study has shown the advantages of femtosecond laser-assisted cataract surgery (FLACS) in terms of patient outcome [4]. When asked in a twin eye study, where one eye had FLACS and the other conventional surgery, patients preferred the conventional approach [5].

Early studies by Nagy and his group had shown the accuracy of the laser capsulotomy [6], but Abell et al. demonstrated why the incidence of capsular tags and tear-out during surgery was higher than in manual CCC [7]. This was due to the femtosecond laser producing a serrated edge, given that it was a pulsed laser. There were also redundant laser spots due to laser spot scatter during the creation of the capsulotomy (Fig. 7.18). This has, to some extent, been resolved by reducing the power in some studies or the vertical spot spacing in others [8] (Fig. 7.19).

However, most surgeons using FLACS say that the laser's most useful function is the way in which it makes the capsulotomy [9]. Might there be other ways to create round, consistently sized capsulotomies?

Another laser, "CAPSULaser" (Excellens, USA), has been under investigation and will soon be available commercially. It is a thermal laser that uses an anterior capsule stained with an optimised solution of trypan blue as its target. Unlike the femtosecond laser, it acts in a continuous manner to create the capsulotomy. The absorption of the laser light, which is in the red/orange part of the spectrum, causes the Type IV collagen in the capsule to change to amorphous collagen. The edge of the capsulotomy is rolled and smooth, and in vitro tests have shown it to be more elastic than that found in manual capsulotomies (Fig. 7.20). Although this is a thermal laser, the time taken to create the capsulotomy is only 1 second, and the overall

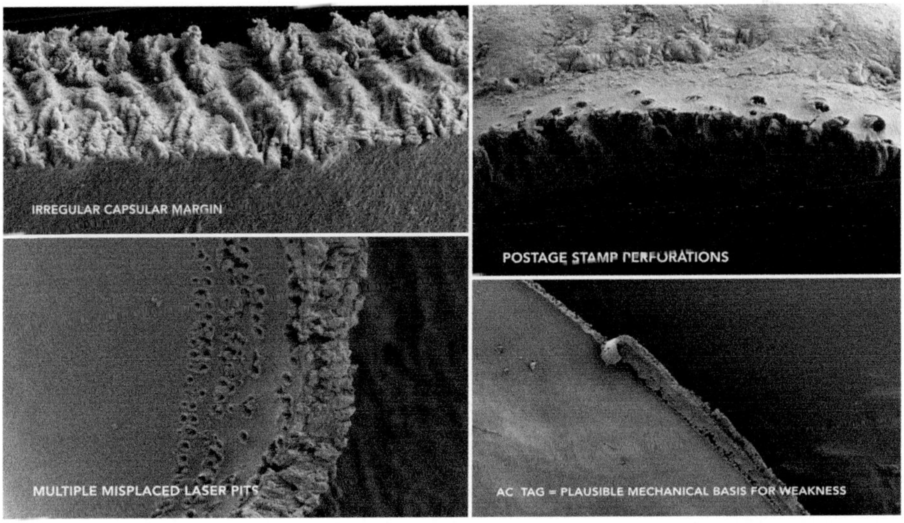

Fig. 7.18 Scanning EM of femtosecond laser capsulotomy edge

Fig. 7.19 Edge of capsulotomy with reduced vertical separation of spots stained with trypan blue

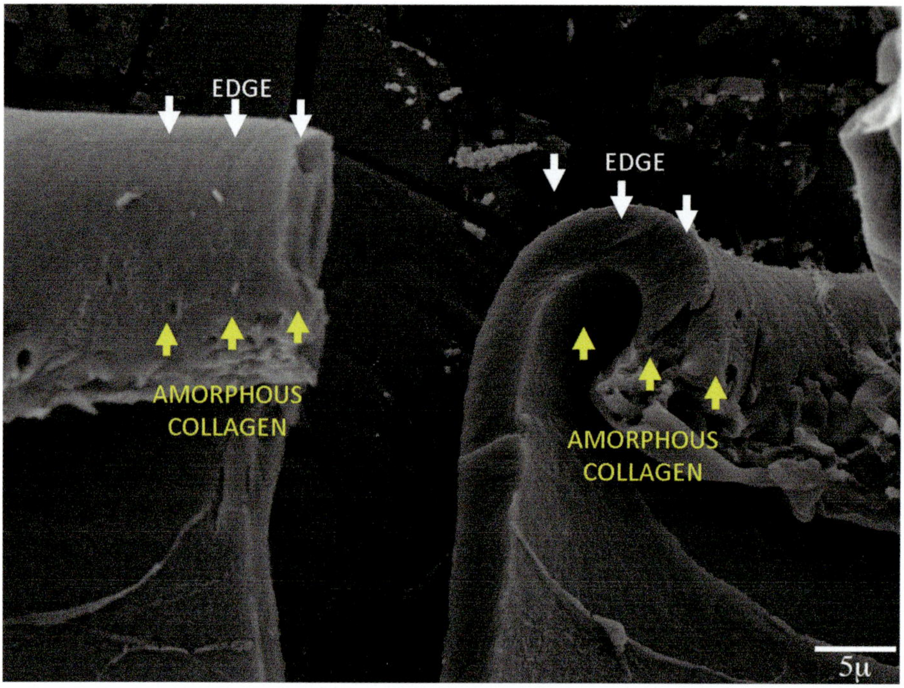

Fig. 7.20 Cut egde of capsulotomy disc made with CAPSULaser

rise in temperature in the anterior chamber is less than 0.2C. The beam is centred by the patient with a fixation light and focused by the surgeon using light sources built into the device. Over 400 human eyes have been studied including, most recently, a CE mark study. This showed a consistency of sizing of 99% within 50 μ of 5 mm (D Mordaunt, P Stodulka, personal communication). Circularity was similarly found. Unlike the femtosecond laser, this device is small and is attached to the underneath of an operating microscope (Fig. 7.21) and does not interfere with the operating

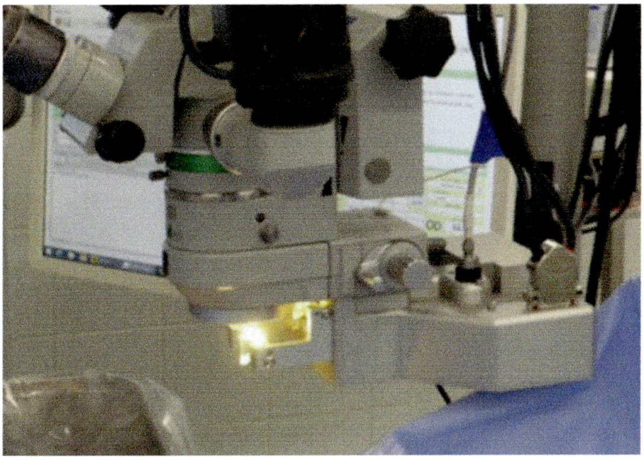

Fig. 7.21 CAPSULaser attached underneath an oprating microscope

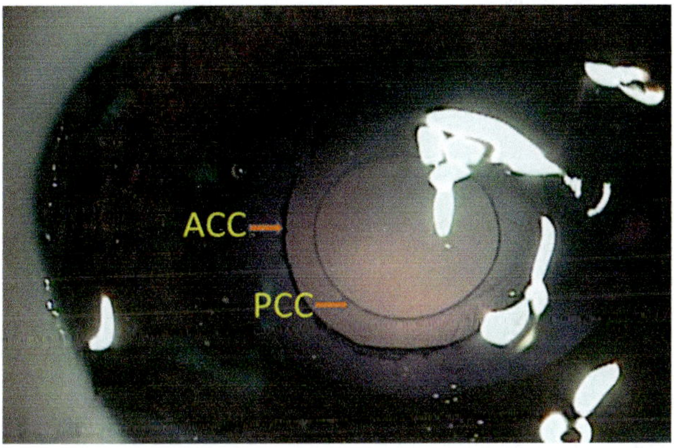

Fig. 7.22 Anterior and posterior capsulotomies in a pig eye made with CAPSULaser

flow. The costs of using this device will be much lower than a femtosecond laser. Given the subject of this book, it is worth noting that posterior capsulotomies have been successfully performed in vitro and human studies will begin soon (Fig. 7.22).

Other thermal devices are also becoming available. A device called "Zepto" is already available in the market, for instance. This consists of a suction ring containing a wire made of nitinol. Nitinol is a metal alloy that has memory, so that when it is deformed, it will return to its original shape. The device, which is single use, is pushed into the eye through the phaco wound, normally 2.5 mm, and is then placed on the anterior capsule. Once it has been centred by the surgeon, suction is applied to attach the device to the capsule (Fig. 7.23). Then a short electrical charge is activated to cut the capsule by causing a phase transition in water molecules with a localised, but small, rise in temperature [10]. This device has also been used in the laboratory for a posterior capsulotomy.

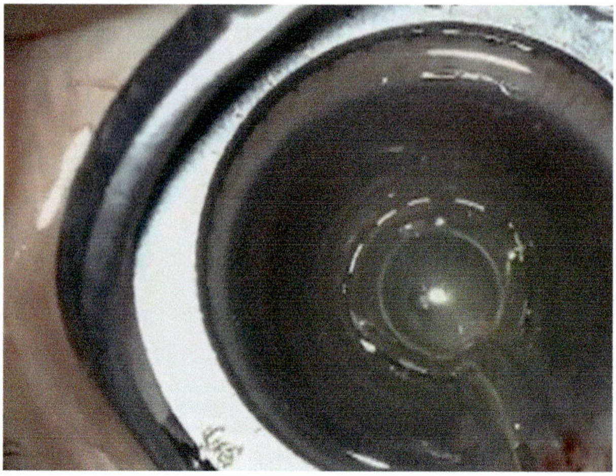

Fig. 7.23 Zepto in position on the anterior capsule

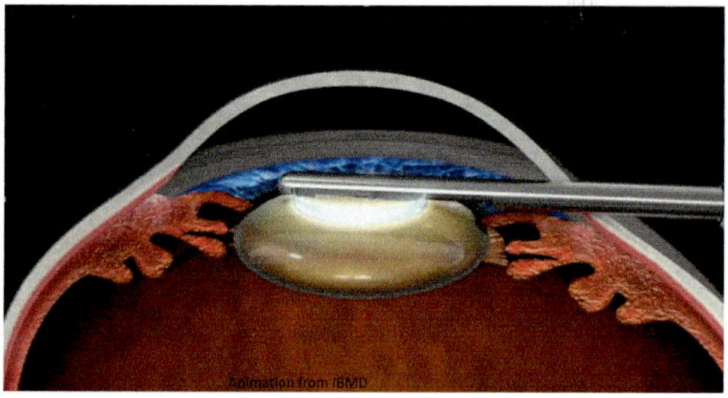

Fig. 7.24 Aperture Rx

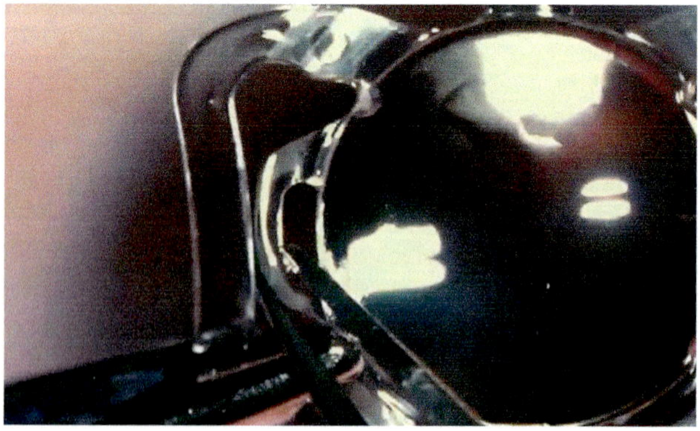

Fig. 7.25 Oculentis Femtis IOL showing anterior mini-haptics

Another not dissimilar approach is that provided by a metal ring that is also pushed into the anterior chamber called “Aperture Rx”. To date, this has not been used on humans. It also acts with localised heat on the anterior capsule to create the capsulotomy (Fig. 7.24).

The anterior capsulotomy has come a long way from its crude beginnings in the eighteenth century. Its role has also changed from allowing access to the lens nucleus, for its expression, to a means of holding an IOL. In this latter role, IOL manufacturers are now realising the possibility of using the perfectly sized and centred capsulotomies created by lasers to hold the IOL in place (Fig. 7.25). It is to be hoped that this will improve refractive outcomes further by making the effective lens position even more predictable.

References

1. Gimbel H, Neuhann T. Development, advantages, and methods of the continuous circular capsulorhexis technique. J Cataract Refract Surg. 1990;16:31–7.
2. Haeussler-Sinangin Y, Dahlhoff D, Schultz T, Dick HB. Clinical performance in continuous curvilinear capsulorhexis creation supported by a digital image guidance system. J Cataract Refract Surg. 2017;43:348–52.
3. Hollick EJ, Spalton DJ, Meacock WR. The effect of capsulorhexis size on posterior capsular opacification: one-year results of a randomized prospective trial. Am J Ophthalmol. 1999;128:271–9.
4. Popovic M, Campos-Muller X, Schlenker M, Ahmed I. Efficacy and safety of femtosecond laser-assisted cataract surgery compared with manual cataract surgery. Ophthalmology. 2016;123(10):2113–26.
5. Mursch-Edlmayr A, Bolz M, Luft N, Ring M, Kreutzer T, Ortner C, Rohleder M, Priglinger S. Intraindividual comparison between femtosecond laser–assisted and conventional cataract surgery. J Cataract Refract Surg. 2017;43(2):215–22.
6. Nagy Z, Takacs A, Filkorn T, Sarayba M. Initial clinical evaluation of an intraocular femtosecond laser in cataract surgery. J Refract Surg. 2009;25:1053–60.
7. Abell RG, Darian-Smith E, Kan JB, Allen PL, Ewe SY, Vote BJ. Femtosecond laser–assisted cataract surgery versus standard phacoemulsification cataract surgery: outcomes and safety in more than 4000 cases at a single center. J Cataract Refract Surg. 2015;41:47–52.
8. Schultz T, Joachim S, Noristani R, Scott W, Dick HB. Greater vertical spot spacing to improve femtosecond laser capsulotomy quality. J Cataract Refract Surg. 2017;3:353–7.
9. Manning S, Barry P, Henry Y, Rosen P, Stenevi U, Young D, Lundström M. Femtosecond laser–assisted cataract surgery versus standard phacoemulsification cataract surgery: study from the European Registry of Quality Outcomes for Cataract and Refractive Surgery. J Cataract Refract Surg. 2016;42:1779–90.
10. Chang DF, Mamalis N, Werner L. Precision pulse capsulotomy; preclinical safety and performance of a new capsulotomy device. Ophthalmology. 2016;123:255–64.

The BIL Anterior Capsulorhexis

8

Sorcha Ní Dhubhghaill and Luc Van Os

8.1 Introduction

The first step in performing a BIL cataract surgery is to perform a well-centered and calibrated anterior continuous curvilinear capsulorhexis (ACCC). A well-implanted BIL relies heavily on the support of the capsule; the anterior capsulorhexis is also a central part of the operation. The ACCC has to fit snugly around the central optic of the lens, and at 5 mm diameter, it is smaller than the typical anterior capsulorhexis [1]. Oversizing the ACCC can result in a lens that is less stable than normal, and this can lead to rotation in the case of toric lenses. If the ACCC is undersized, then lens insertion can be more difficult and can result in zonular trauma. In this chapter, we describe the ACCC technique that we use to facilitate a bag-in-the-lens intraocular implant.

8.2 Indications

All modern cataract surgeries require an ACCC, but since the BIL is a capsular-supported lens, it requires an adaptation to the standard technique. The anterior capsular opening required to accommodate the optic of the BIL implant is 5 mm, which is slightly smaller than the standard "in-the-bag" technique. Subsequently, the anterior rhexis becomes the guide for the primary posterior capsulorhexis (Chap. 7). Creating too large a capsulorhexis will risk lens instability and lens prolapse, too

Electronic Supplementary Material The online version of this chapter (https://doi.org/10.1007/978-3-030-03086-5_8) contains supplementary material, which is available to authorized users.

S. Ní Dhubhghaill (✉) · L. Van Os
Department of Ophthalmology, Antwerp University, University Hospital, Edegem, Belgium
e-mail: sorcha.nidhubhghaill@uza.be

M.-J. Tassignon et al. (eds.), *Innovative Implantation Technique*,
https://doi.org/10.1007/978-3-030-03086-5_8

small a capsulorhexis and the insertion of the lens is difficult and can stress the zonular suspension excessively. Femtosecond laser surgical technology can be used to create the optimal capsulorhexis, but we can also achieve a similar result through the use of a ring caliper device [2, 3]. The ring caliper is made from a material called PEMA which retains a memory of its shape. It can be injected through incisions as small as 1.2 mm and still returns to its original shape once inside the eye. The ring is available in both a 5 mm and 4.5 mm, for adults and children, respectively.

8.3 Surgical Technique

The anterior chamber is prepared by filling it with an ophthalmic viscosurgical device (OVD). We use both a k-hook ring inserter and a suture-tying forceps to place the ring. The posterior edge of the ring is grasped with the forceps to stabilize it, and it is led into the anterior chamber with the anterior notch of the k-hook at the anterior edge. Exerting a small amount of posterior tension with the forceps stretches the ring into a thinner, oblong shape and makes it easier to insert (Fig. 8.1).

Once the ring is halfway through the incision, the forceps can be released and the k-hook can complete the insertion alone. The ring is then pushed down onto the lens capsule. If the ring remains loose and suspended in the anterior chamber, then it will not remain stable during the capsulorhexis and will provide no guidance for the ACCC. We secure it by using the inferior notch of the k-hook inserter to push it onto the anterior capsule (Fig. 8.2).

The BIL is one of the few lenses for which the surgeon can determine exactly where they want to place the lens, and, as such, great care must be taken to align the lens correctly. There is currently some debate as to how to achieve the best

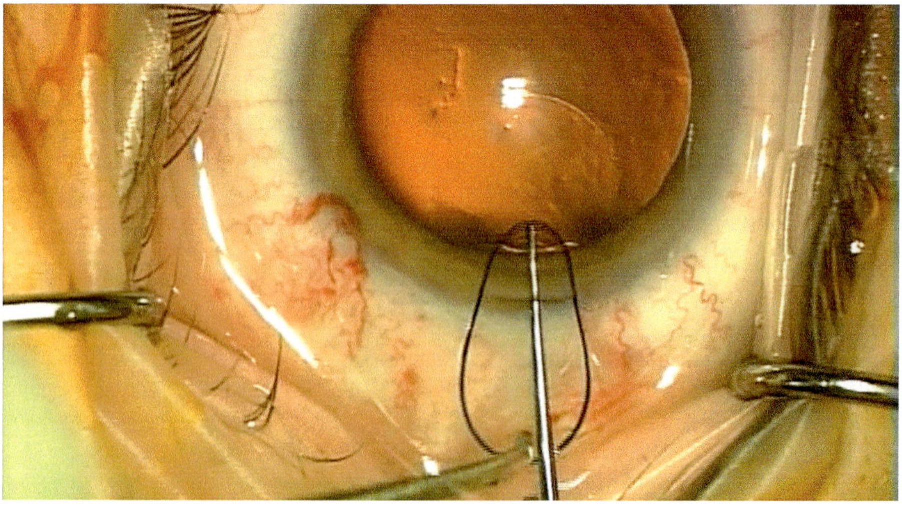

Fig. 8.1 Insertion of the ring caliper using forceps and a k-hook

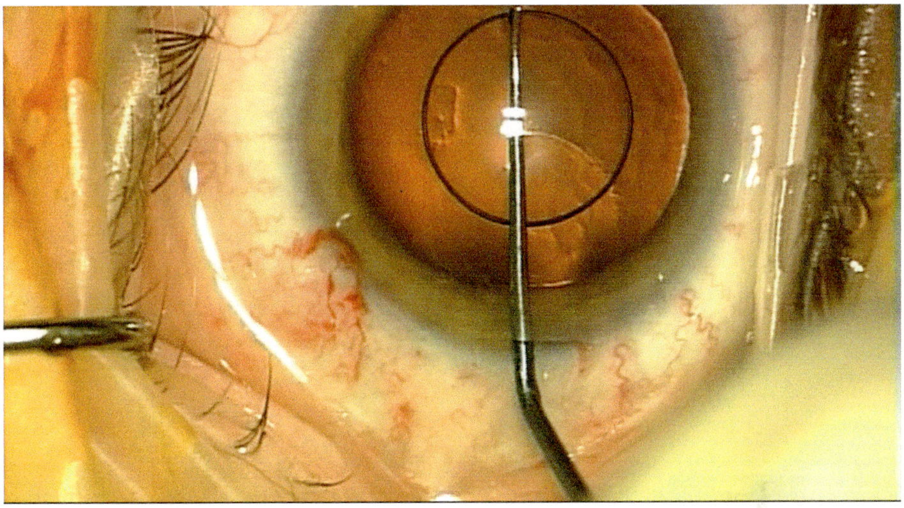

Fig. 8.2 Positioning the ring caliper onto the anterior capsule

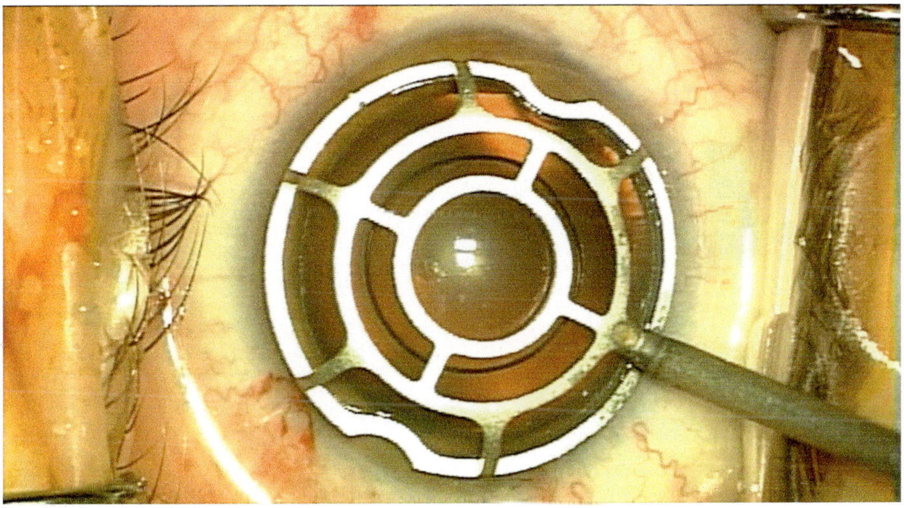

Fig. 8.3 Eye Cage device with P1 and the ring caliper visible centrally

centration. We use a combination of an Eye Cage device (Fig. 8.3), the Purkinje (Purkinje-Sanson) light reflexes, and the corneoscleral limbus.

Four Purkinje images are usually visible in a normal eye. The first (P1) can be seen from the outer surface of the cornea, and the second (P2) can be seen from the inner surface of the cornea. The third (P3) can be viewed from the anterior lens,

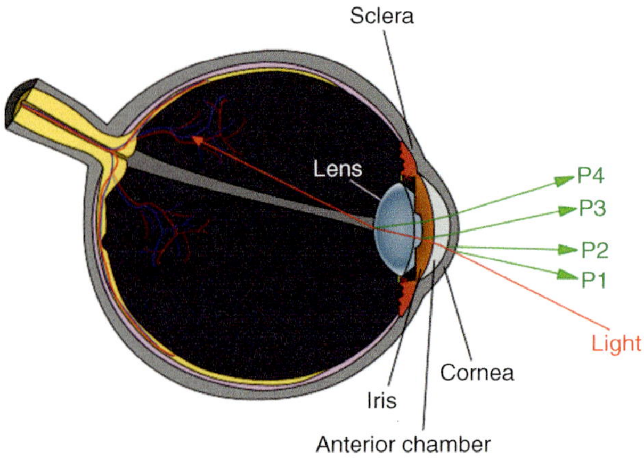

Fig. 8.4 Source of the Purkinje light reflexes

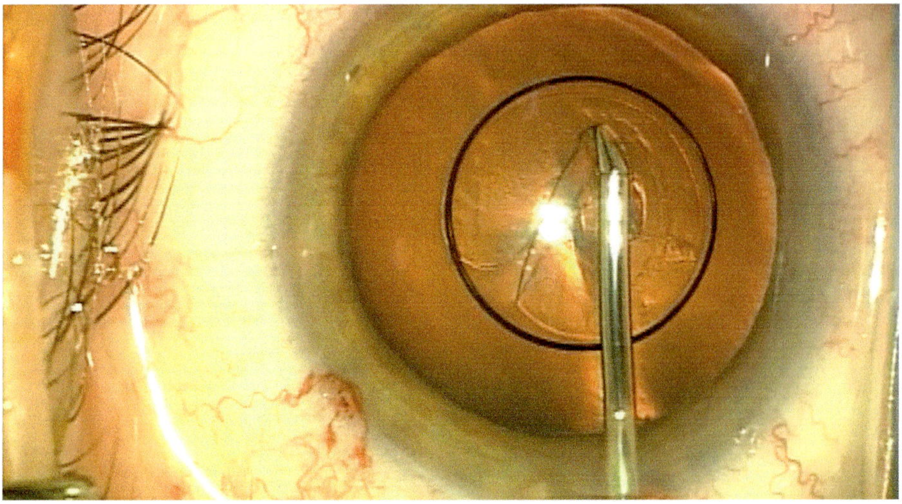

Fig. 8.5 Performing the ACCC in the center of the ring caliper

while the fourth (P4) can be seen through the reflection from the posterior surface of the lens. The fourth, unlike the other three images, is inverted (Fig. 8.4).

In general, we perform the technique under topical anesthesia so that the patient can be asked to fixate on a target. Then we use P1 and P4, as well as the corneoscleral limbus, to center the Eye Cage device. If the ring caliper is not well-centered, then the tip of the OVD cannula can be used to nudge the ring over the capsule and into position. Once the ring is in the correct position, then we inject OVD in a circle over the ring to lock it in place to prevent movement during the subsequent steps.

The ACCC can then be performed by using the surgeon's own preferred technique. We use a microforceps to perform the rhexis, taking care to remain inside the guidance of the ring caliper (Fig. 8.5). Once the capsulorhexis is completed, we use the close tip of the microforceps to lift the ring off of the capsule and then grasp it. As we remove the ring, we also rotate the forceps to ease the ring's removal. The phacoemulsification can then be continued as normal.

8.4 Complications

If the capsulorhexis is too small, then it is very difficult to insert the lens without stretching the capsular bag and damaging the zonules. In these cases, it is best to restart the rhexis and to widen it before proceeding. If the rhexis either runs out or is too large, then a BIL can still be placed; however, the PPCCC must be the correct size to support the lens. If there is a posterior capsular tear during the phacoemulsification, a BIL can still be implanted that is just supported by the ACCC and, thus, ensuring a perfect fit is essential. It is best to slightly undersize the capsulorhexis for a toric BIL, so as to ensure a very secure fit around the lens. If the rhexis is loose, it can lead to a rotation of the lens, and the corrective toric effect can be lost [4]. If the ACCC is too large to support the BIL and the PPCCC is not sufficient, the next step is to use Bean-shaped ring segments to support the lens. The Bean-shaped ring segment technique is described elsewhere (Chap. 16).

8.5 Core Messages

- Prepare your capsule by filling the anterior chamber and by flattening the capsule.
- Always use a ring caliper to ensure that the size and centration of the rhexis are correct.
- Check the position of the ring with an Eye Cage device.
- Stabilize or "lock" the ring on the surface anterior capsule to prevent slipping.
- Widen the ACCC if it is too small.

8.6 Instruments Used

The instruments listed are our preference, but similar ones can be used based on the surgeon's own preference.

Item	Description	Manufacturer
OVD	Healon, Healon GV	Abbott Medical Optics, USA
IOL rotator	Spatula	Bausch & Lomb
Rycroft	OVD cannula	Steriseal, included in OVD package
Microforceps	Ikeda angled 30° Capsulorhexis 23.0 g forceps	EyeTech Fr2268
Ring caliper	PMMA ring with a 4.5 mm or 5 mm inner diameter	Type 4 L, 5, Morcher, Germany

References

1. Gimbel H, Neuhann T. Developments, advantages, and methods of the continuous circular capsulorhexis technique. J Cataract Refract Surg. 1990;16:31–7.
2. Tassignon M, Rozema JJ, Gobin L. Ring-shaped caliper for better anterior capsulorhexis sizing and centration. J Cataract Refract Surg. 2006;32:1253–5.
3. Ni Dhubhghaill STM, Tassignon MJ. Regarding the open ring-shaped guider for a continuous curvilinear capsulorhexis. J Cataract Refract Surg. 2015;41:2592.
4. Tassignon M, Gobin L. Toric bag-in-the-lens implant: why and how to implant. Expert Rev Ophthalmol. 2010;5:135–41.

The Posterior Capsulorhexis

9

Sorcha Ní Dhubhghaill

9.1 Introduction

The lens capsule is produced by lens epithelial cells (LECs) and is the thickest basement membrane found in the body. The thickness of the capsule is not uniform and is thinner on the posterior surface than on the anterior. The posterior capsule can be as thin as 9 microns in some regions, far thinner than its anterior counterpart [1]. The capsule is composed of a membrane-like collagen structure that, separates the anterior from the posterior segments. Resident surgeons in their training years are taught to be very cautious and to guard the posterior capsule as accidental rupture of the posterior capsule is known to be associated with higher rates of postoperative complications [2]. Gimbal and Neuhann first described a technique for removing a central region of the posterior capsule as a means for preventing posterior capsular opacification (PCO) in high-risk cases [3]. While accidental posterior capsular rupture is associated with vitreous loss and damage to the anterior hyaloid face, a planned and well-controlled primary posterior continuous curvilinear capsulorhexis (PPCCC) can be just as safe as operating with an intact capsule [4–6].

9.2 Indications for a PPCCC

The PPCCC is an essential step in the BIL surgical technique. However, it can also be applied to other situations too, such as in pediatric cataract and uveitis and for optic buttonholing [7, 8], and to repair accidental capsular ruptures [3]. It should be

Electronic Supplementary Material The online version of this chapter (https://doi.org/10.1007/978-3-030-03086-5_9) contains supplementary material, which is available to authorized users.

S. Ní Dhubhghaill (✉)
Department of Ophthalmology, Antwerp University, University Hospital, Edegem, Belgium
e-mail: sorcha.nidhubhghaill@uza.be

M.-J. Tassignon et al. (eds.), *Innovative Implantation Technique*,
https://doi.org/10.1007/978-3-030-03086-5_9

noted that while PPCCC can be used to reduce the rate of PCO in high-risk cases, it does not eradicate PCO completely. The rate of visual axis reopacification in elderly patients can be up to 2% after 2 years [9], and 23–40% can experience partial or complete closure of the posterior capsulorhexis [10, 11] in high-risk cases such as pediatric cataract or uveitis. A PPCCC alone is, therefore, insufficient to preventing PCO in the long term. The BIL implant is the only lens that requires a PPCCC for implantation, and, given that it is our standard lens, we perform PPCCCs hundreds of times each year. Based on our experience, we have developed a standardized approach which is described in this chapter (Fig. 9.1).

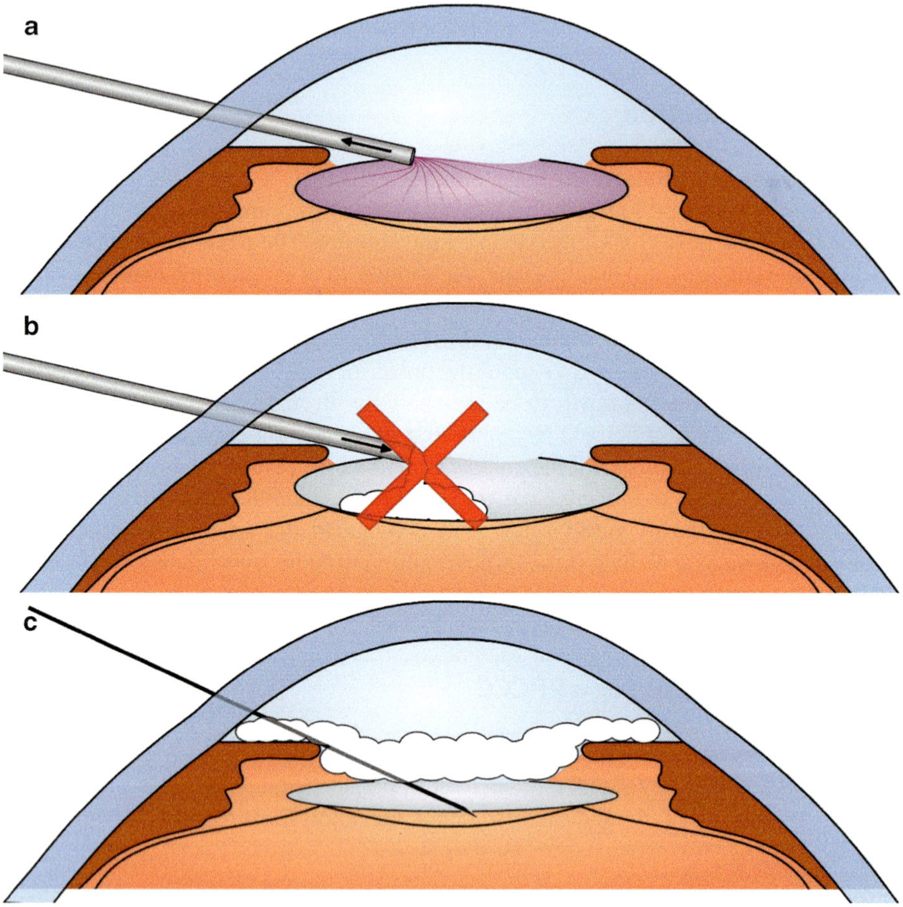

Fig. 9.1 PPCCC step-by-step schematic

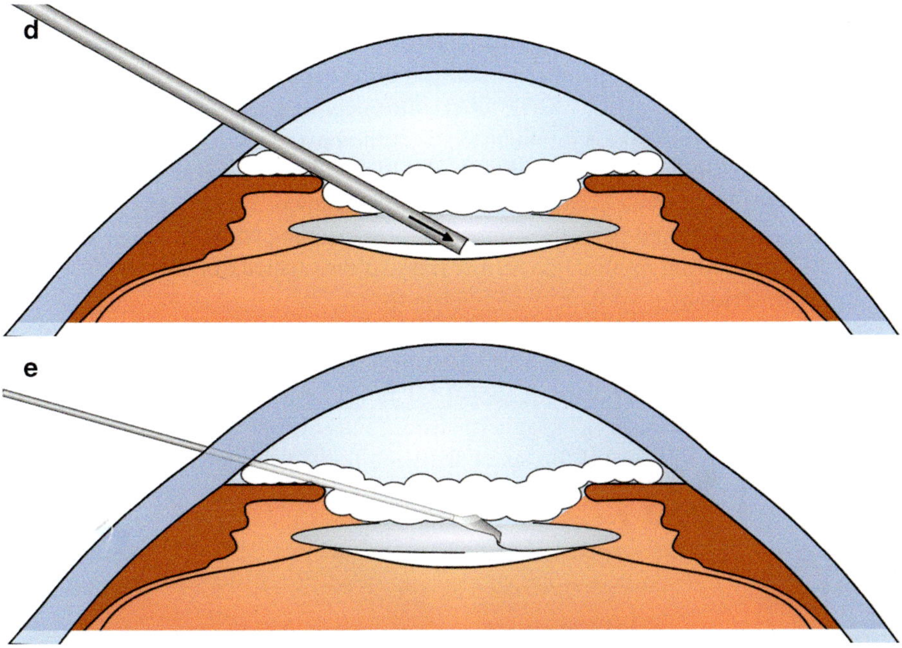

Fig. 9.1 (continued)

9.3 Surgical Technique

Firstly, the anterior capsulorhexis is performed as described previously (Chap. 8). The ring of the anterior rhexis is used to determine the correct dimensions of the PPCCC without the need for the ring caliper's reinsertion. The cataract may be removed using the surgeon's preferred technique, but it should be noted that the ACCC is smaller in the BIL technique than it is in the standard lens-in-bag surgery; surgeons who use a chopping technique should bear this in mind. Once the lens nucleus and residual lens cortex have been removed, an ophthalmic viscosurgical device (OVD) is used to refill the anterior chamber but not the capsular bag - this is important.

We prefer to use a cohesive OVD (Healon GV; Abbott Medical Optics, USA) for various reasons. The injection should be performed over the plane of the iris so that it is compressing and flattening the anterior chamber while also refilling the eye. The goal here is to bring the anterior and posterior capsules together to make the lens implantation easier. Injecting OVD in a ring "donut shape" over the level of the iris can also express residual fluid out of the capsular bag, through the anterior capsular opening. It also counteracts the posterior pressure, flattening the capsule, which is the optimal shape for performing a PPCCC. It is essential that no OVD be injected into the bag itself; filling the bag with OVD pushes the posterior capsule downwards and into a concave shape, making the process more difficult and less predictable when performing the PPCCC.

The next step is to aspirate any residual lens fibers and fluid from the bag using a Helsinki cannula (1273E Steriseal Video 9.1). This step ensures that there is no OVD in the bag and that the anterior and posterior capsules are in apposition. The PPCCC starts with a small (30G or tuberculin) needle, used to create an opening (Fig. 9.2a). Be sure to take a moment to select the best place for the puncture, one that is easy to visualize, not obscured by the light reflexes, and not too peripheral and that will be the most comfortable for the subsequent rhexis hand maneuvers. The puncture should be performed in a lateral scratching motion, rather than in a downward puncturing motion; the former reduces the chance of inadvertently puncturing the anterior hyaloid face.

For the next step, we use a low-molecular-weight cohesive OVD (regular Healon OVD; Abbott Medical Optics, USA) with a Rycroft cannula, threading it through the small opening in the posterior capsule. The OVD is injected into the space of Berger. It typically starts as a "spaghetti string," but it forms a more cohesive "blister" shape as it comes to fill the space between the capsule and anterior hyaloid.

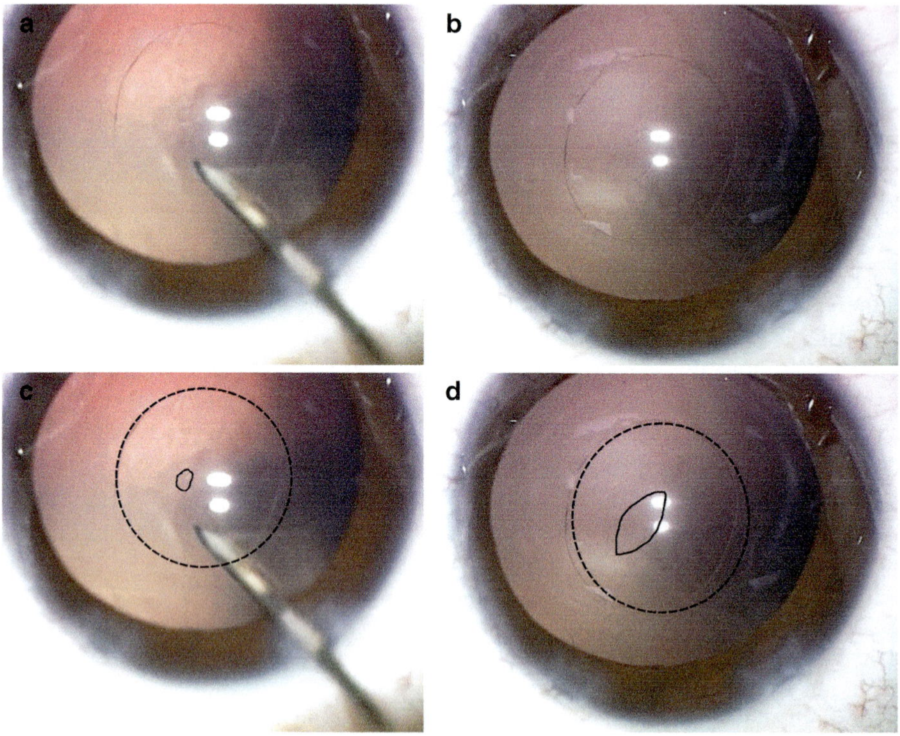

Fig. 9.2 Performing the puncture (**a**, **c**) and observing the widening "split" (**b**, **d**)

The cushion OVD should be increased until it is slightly larger than the ACCC, thereby acting as a tamponade to possible vitreous loss. At this point, the small capsular opening will usually split open (Fig. 9.2b). The split's size should be kept to one that is smaller than the ACCC. The surgeon must, therefore, be very focused when performing this step. This split is usually accompanied by a smooth edge and an edge with a flap. We use an Ikeda microforceps (Fr2268 EyeTech) to grasp the flap to perform the rhexis and match the dimensions of the anterior rhexis. With time, and through repeating the exercise, the surgeon will come to develop a feel for how and where the capsule will split during the OVD injection. This can be used to personalize the technique to each individual surgeon's most comfortable hand position.

9.4 Complications

If the PPCCC is undersized, then inserting the lens can be difficult and can result in extra zonular stress. Extra effort should be taken, therefore, to widen small PPCCCs. We recommend using straight microscissors or back-cut microscissors to restart the rhexis, depending on the shape of the opening. We do not advise using the needle again because the position required to cut the capsule is too vertical and could inadvertently disturb the anterior vitreous. Once a small cut has been made, we use the microforceps to lift the flap and to widen the opening along an arc, thereby increasing the size of the aperture. Once it is wide enough, the flap is pulled centrally to complete, and to restore, the continuous curvilinear shape.

In cases of zonular instability, the lack of counter traction makes the PPCCC more complex and less predictable. In these cases, we use a capsular tension ring (CTR) to provide the necessary counter traction. The sizing of the CTR is very important; too small a size will provide little counter traction, too large a size will stretch the capsule like a drumhead, and the PPCCC puncture may elicit a very large capsule tear, rather than a small and discrete puncture. We generally select a CTR 1–2 mm smaller than the white-to-white measurement, which most often corresponds to an 11 mm CTR. We also recommend the routine insertion of a CTR in patients with an axial length ≥26.0 mm because larger eyes tend to have larger capsules, requiring additional stabilization to prevent wobbling of the BIL.

If the ACCC is larger than the normal 5 mm, or in cases of lens exchange for which the ACCC is irregular, the creation of the PPCCC requires the insertion of the ring caliper for size and centration. In these cases, the ring is inserted as described previously and rested on top of the anterior/posterior capsule complex; it is removed once the PPCCC is complete (Fig. 9.3).

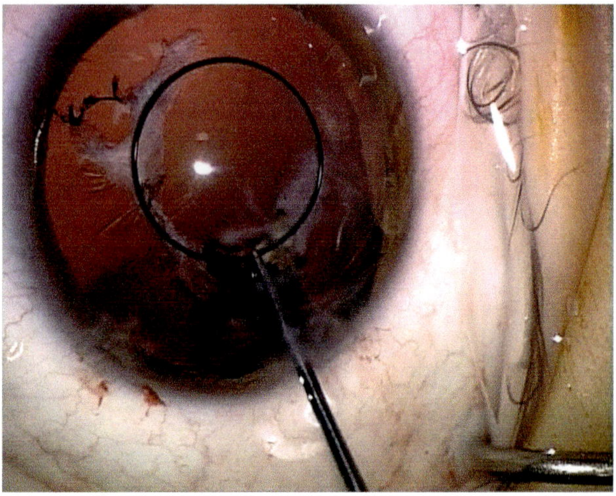

Fig. 9.3 Using the ring caliper to perform the PPCCC in a post trauma case

9.5 Core Messages

- Prepare your capsule by filling the anterior chamber and flattening the capsule.
- Do not fill the capsule with OVD.
- Do not puncture downward; use a lateral movement instead.
- Observe how the OVD collects in the space of Berger.
- Widen the PPCCC if it is too small.
- Use a CTR to provide a more stable bag, if necessary.
- If your ACCC is not the correct size or shape, then the ring caliper can be used to provide the correct sizing of the PPCCC.

9.6 Instruments Used

The instruments listed below are our preferred instruments, but similar ones can be used based upon the surgeon's individual preference.

Item	Description	Manufacturer
OVD	Healon, Healon GV	Abbott Medical Optics, USA
Helsinki	Aspiration cannula	Hurricane Medical, Steriseal 1273E
Rycroft	OVD cannula	Steriseal, included in OVD package
Microforceps	Ikeda angled 30° Capsulorhexis 23.0 g forceps	EyeTech Fr2268
Microscissors straight	Straight scissors, curved shaft	EyeTech Fr2275
Microscissors back cut	23G scissor 45°	EyeTech VR1514
Capsular tension ring	PMMA 11–13 mm	Type 14C Morcher, Germany

References

1. Barraquer R, Michael R, Abreu R, Lamarca J, Tresserra F. Human lens capsule thickness as a function of age and location along the sagittal lens perimeter. Invest Ophthalmol Vis Sci. 2006;47:2053.
2. Vajpayee R, Sharma N, Dada T, Gupta V, Kumar A, Dada VK. Management of posterior capsule tears. Surv Ophthalmol. 2001;45:473–88.
3. Gimbel H, Neuhann T. Developments, advantages, and methods of the continuous circular capsulorhexis technique. J Cataract Refract Surg. 1990;16:31–7.
4. DeGroot V, Hubert M, VanBest JA, Engelen S, Vab Aelst S, Tassignon MJ. Lack of fluorophotometric evidence of aqueous-vitreous barrier disruption after posterior capsulorhexis. J Cataract Refract Surg. 2003;29:2330–8.
5. Leysen I, Coeckelbergh T, Gobin L, Smet H, Daniel Y, DeGroot V, Tassignon MJ. Cumulative neodymium: YAG laser rates after bag-in-the-lens and lens-in-the-bag intraocular lens implantation: comparative study. J Cataract Refract Surg. 2006;32:2085–90.
6. Menapace R. Posterior capsulorhexis combined with optic buttonholing: an alternative to standard in-the-bag implantation of sharp-edged intraocular lenses? A critical analysis of 1000 consecutive cases. Graefes Arch Clin Exp Ophthalmol. 2008;246:787–801.
7. Gimbel H, DeBroff BM. Posterior capsulorhexis with optic capture: maintaining a clear visual axis after pediatric cataract surgery. J Cataract Refract Surg. 1994;20:658.
8. Gimbel H. Posterior continuous curvilinear capsulorhexis and optic capture of the intraocular lens to prevent secondary opacification in pediatric cataract surgery. J Cataract Refract Surg. 1997;23:652–6.
9. Yazici A, Bozkurt E, Kara N, Yildirim Y, Demirok A, Yilmaz OF. Long-term results of phacoemulsification combined with primary posterior curvilinear capsulorhexis in adults. Mid East Af. J Ophthalmol. 2012;19:115–9.
10. Tassignon M, DeGroot V, Smets RM, Tawab B, Vervecken F. Secondary closure of posterior continuous curvilinear capsulorhexis. J Cataract Refract Surg. 1996;22:1200–9.
11. Tassignon M, DeGroot V, Vervecken F, Van Tenten Y. Secondary closure of posterior continuous curvilinear capsulorhexis in normal eyes and eyes at risk for postoperative inflammation. J Cataract Refract Surg. 1998;24:1333–8.

Lens Preparation and Folding

10

Sorcha Ní Dhubhghaill

10.1 Introduction

Once the matching anterior and posterior capsulorhexes are complete, the next step is to prepare and to fold the lens implant. The BIL implant is an acrylic hydrophilic lens with a 28% water content making it a very flexible lens [1]. The total diameter of the lens, from haptic to haptic, is 7.5 mm [2]. The central optic diameter is 5 mm. The lenses are available as standard from 10.0D to 30.0D in 0.5 diopter increments, but other powers as well as toric versions are available upon request. Toric corrections are also available on request. A preloaded injection system is not yet on the market, so the lens must be folded manually. In this chapter, we describe our technique for lens preparation and folding.

10.2 Surgical Technique

We use a non-toothed suture-tying forceps to lift the lens out of the lens packaging. Care should be taken not to touch the central optic, because the lens is made out of a hydrophilic material and any contact can reduce the quality of the implant. The lens is lifted by the haptic groove as shown below (Fig. 10.1).

There are currently two injection systems used for BIL implantation, both available from Medicel. The standard injector (Medicel ACCUJECT 2.5-3P LP604540) can be used for all diopters, but it does require a 2.8 mm incision for implantation. This system comes in two pieces, the injector and a loading unit. The IOL is dropped onto the loading unit and is aligned with the anterior haptic horizontally and the posterior haptic vertically (Fig. 10.2). For a non-toric lens implant, there is no difference between the anterior or posterior surfaces; thus, it is not possible to place it

S. Ní Dhubhghaill (✉)
Department of Ophthalmology, Antwerp University, University Hospital, Edegem, Belgium
e-mail: sorcha.nidhubhghaill@uza.be

M.-J. Tassignon et al. (eds.), *Innovative Implantation Technique*,
https://doi.org/10.1007/978-3-030-03086-5_10

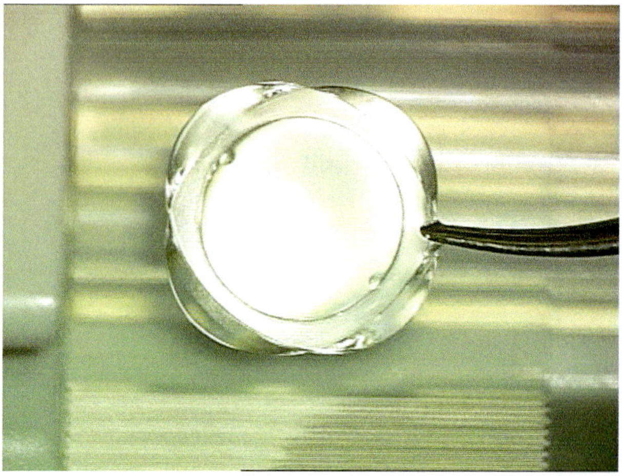

Fig. 10.1 Lifting a toric BIL implant by the haptic edge

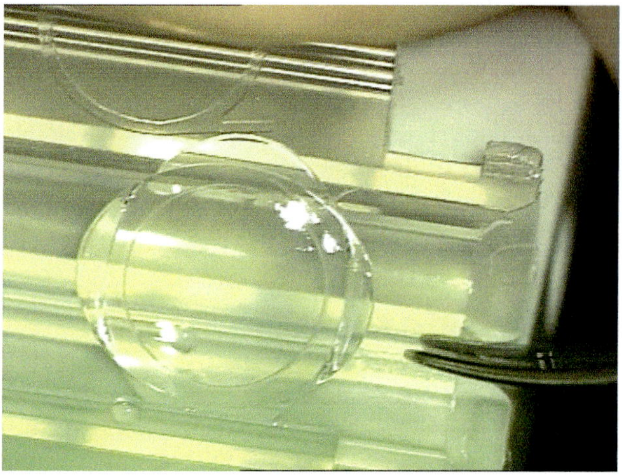

Fig. 10.2 Placing the lens on the loading unit

upside-down. Toric lenses must have their toric alignment markers anteriorly prior to loading so care must be taken to check the lens before the loading and folding. This cannot be done with the naked eye and should be done under microscope guidance (Fig. 10.3). The newer Medical injectors are one-piece systems that are available for smaller incisions. In general, I use a 2.2 mm injector for lens diopters of 24 or less. Between 24 and 26 diopters, I use a 2.6 mm, and for 27 diopters and above, I inject the lens through a 2.8 mm incision. The tip of the injector is more angled than the previous generation of injectors, so you have to be careful that the lens is not injected too deeply. Be sure to angle the injector so that the lens opens in the anterior chamber, above the bag. If you find that the lens tends to dive too deeply, you can you a side port instrument in your non-dominant had while you inject, as a barrier to guide the lens in the anterior chamber.

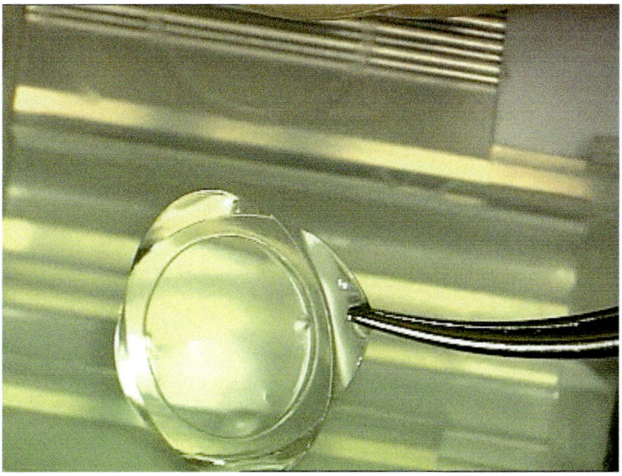

Fig. 10.3 Tilting the toric lens to confirm the anterior location of the toric marking

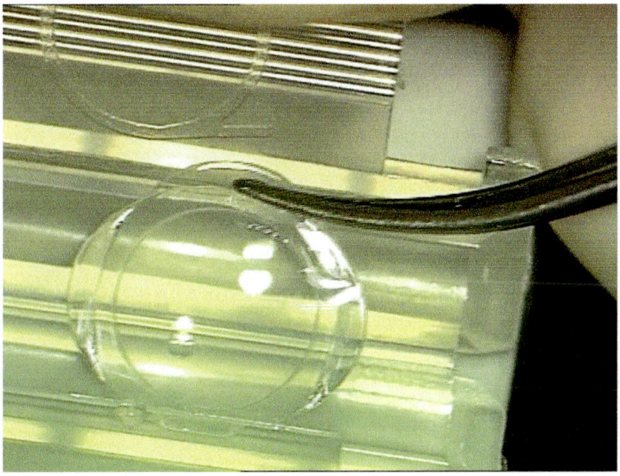

Fig. 10.4 Tucking the posterior haptics into the loading unit

Aligning the posterior haptics vertically puts them in the best position to tuck it under the ridge of the loading unit with the suture-tying forceps (Fig. 10.4).

Ensuring that the haptics are well tucked into the cartridge makes the folding of the lens more secure. Once the lens is in place, the cartridge can be filled with OVD (Fig. 10.5), and the lens is ready to be folded. Lower-diopter, thinner lenses are easier to fold than the higher diopters. When folding the lens, a useful tip is to observe the folding from the side so that you can better see that the lens is folding into the cartridge in the correct direction. Occasionally, the lens can fold in the opposite direction; forcing the fold can damage the lens.

Once the lens has been folded, the cartridge is inserted into the injector and locked into place. The blue plunger is advanced into the cartridge and the lens is pushed into the tip of the injector. The lens can be seen folding into a roll as it is advanced towards the tip (Fig. 10.6).

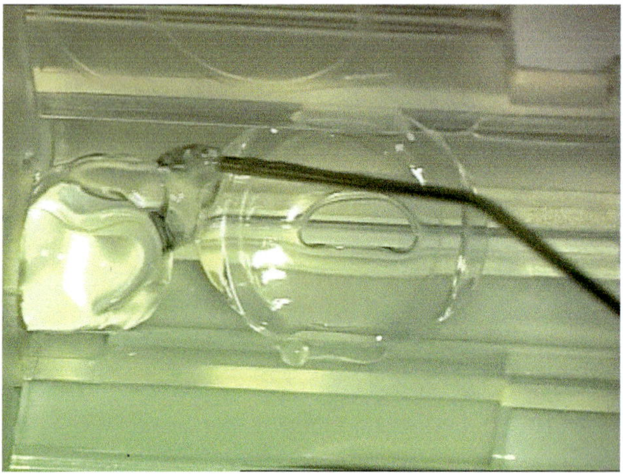

Fig. 10.5 Coating the lens and filling the cartridge with OVD

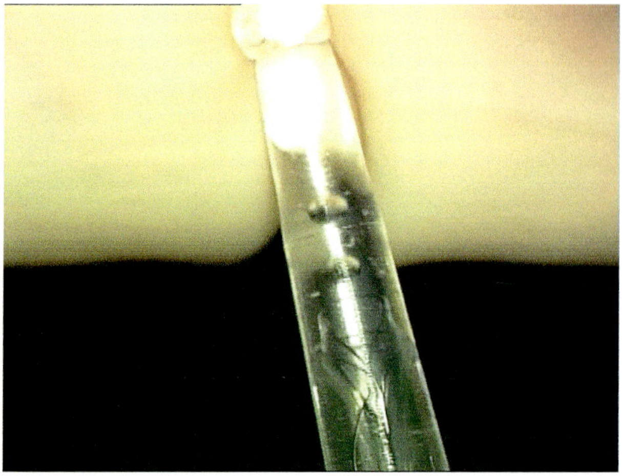

Fig. 10.6 Advancing the lens to the tip of the injector

Since the anterior chamber has already been filled with OVD during the PPCCC, we empty the extra OVD out of the cartridge prior to injection. The second lens injection system is the ACCUJECT 2.2-1P (LP604540). These injectors are a one-piece system with the cartridge already attached to the injector. The lens is dropped onto the loading area, aligned as previously (Fig. 10.2) and is then slid under the plastic cover with a tying forceps. It can then be folded and prepared for injection.

10.3 Complications

Occasionally, the haptics can be folded during the injection process. This appears as a ripple in the haptics of the BIL and if it occurs, the groove is closed off and the implant cannot be implanted in the capsular opening. The solution in this case is to hold one of the haptic's flanges to stabilize the lens and to use a second instrument to open the groove. We tend to use a blunt IOL rotator (Bausch and Lomb), and once the tip of the instrument enters the groove, you can see a popping action as the haptics return to their normal position. The lens can now be inserted as normal.

10.4 Core Messages

- Never touch the central optic when manipulating the lens; lift the lens by the peripheral haptic edge.
- Ensure that there is plenty of OVD in the lens cartridge to lubricate the lens folding and injection.
- Become familiar with the feel of folding the lens. There should be some mild resistance with lower-power lenses folding more easily than higher-power ones.
- If the resistance is too high, do not force the lens to fold, given that it is likely in the wrong position. Recheck the lens placement in the cartridge, add more OVD and try folding the lens again.
- Angle the injector to ensure that the lens opens over the bag and doesn't dive into the vitreous. A side-port instrument can help.

10.5 Instruments Used

The instruments listed below are our preferences, but similar ones can be used based on the surgeon's preference.

Item	Description	Manufacturer
OVD	Healon, Healon GV	Abbott Medical Optics, USA
2.8 mm injector	Two-piece injection set	ACCUJECT 2.5-3P LP604540, Medicel, Switzerland
2.2 mm to 2.6 mm injector	One-piece injection set	ACCUJECT 2.2-1P LP604500, Medicel, Switzerland
Microforceps	Ikeda angled 30° Capsulorhexis 23.0 g forceps	EyeTech Fr2268

References

1. Tassignon M, Gobin L, Mathysen D, Van Looveren J, De Groot V. Clinical outcomes of cataract surgery after bag-in-the-lens intraocular lens implantation following ISO standard 11979-7:2006. J Cataract Refract Surg. 2011;37:2120–9.
2. Tassignon M, Gobin L, Mathysen D, Van Looveren J, DeGroot V. Clinical outcomes of cataract surgery after the bag in-the-lens intraocular lens implantation following ISO standard 11979-7. J Cataract Refract Surg. 2006;37:2120–9.

BIL Lens Insertion

11

Sorcha Ní Dhubhghaill

11.1 Introduction

The BIL insertion technique differs from that of standard lenses. While most lenses can be injected directly into the capsular bag, the BIL requires a two-step approach. The key to safe BIL cataract surgery is to always respect and preserve the anterior hyaloid face. Disrupting the face can result in complications such as cystoid macular edema and retinal detachment, while maintaining an intact vitreous makes BIL cataract surgery just as safe as the standard lens in the capsular bag approach, with all the additional BIL benefits.

11.2 Lens Insertion

The BIL can be injected through wounds as small as 2 mm, depending on the surgeon's preference and the refractive power of the implant. The larger lenses (>28 dioptre spherical power) can be prone to damage if squeezed through a small wound and should be injected though larger, 2.6 mm incisions. In this chapter, we describe our approach to the safe injection and placement of the BIL implant.

Electronic Supplementary Material The online version of this chapter (https://doi.org/10.1007/978-3-030-03086-5_11) contains supplementary material, which is available to authorized users.

S. Ní Dhubhghaill (✉)
Department of Ophthalmology, Antwerp University, University Hospital, Edegem, Belgium
e-mail: sorcha.nidhubhghaill@uza.be

M.-J. Tassignon et al. (eds.), *Innovative Implantation Technique*,
https://doi.org/10.1007/978-3-030-03086-5_11

11.3 Surgical Technique

The lens is slowly injected into the anterior chamber. Aim to inject the lens over the anterior capsule and not directly into position. Trying to inject the lens immediately into the two capsulorhexes is more uncontrolled and runs the risk of causing vitreous prolapse. We therefore break down the lens insertion into two steps. The first step is to inject the lens into that anterior chamber over the level of the iris, by holding the injector at a low angle (Fig. 11.1). If you find that the lenses tend to inject too deeply and dive through the posterior rhexis you can use a side port instrument in your non-dominant hand to guide the IOL and keep it horizontal and in the anterior chamber.

Once the lens unfolds, any cellular material or blood behind the lens can be aspirated using a Helsinki cannula. Taking this step ensures that there will be no material behind the lens after insertion because there is no method of removing it. After cleaning any retrolenticular haze, the lens is then pushed down on top of the anterior capsule by injecting a cushion of OVD over the lens. This not only stabilizes the lens for insertion, but it also provides another moment where the anterior and posterior capsules can be pushed together to ease insertion (Fig. 11.2). The biggest obstacle to simple lens implantation is the separation of the two capsular layers.

Inserting the lens starts by tilting the posterior haptic under the posterior capsule and pushing laterally, placing both capsules in the lens groove (Fig. 11.3). This step starts the process of capturing the capsules in the groove. During this movement, the cushion of OVD behind the lens will start to move toward the anterior chamber, thereby reducing the amount of OVD in the space of Berger, but the vitreous does not typically follow.

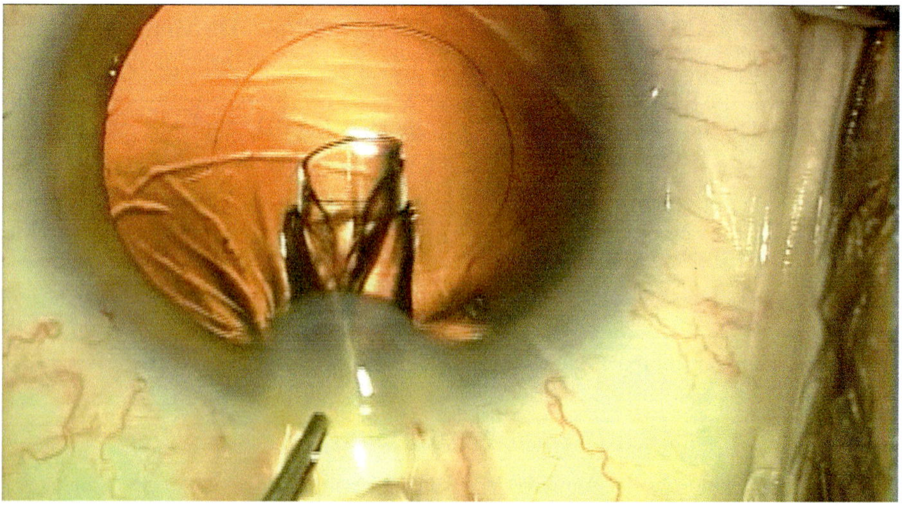

Fig. 11.1 Controlled injection of the lens into the anterior chamber

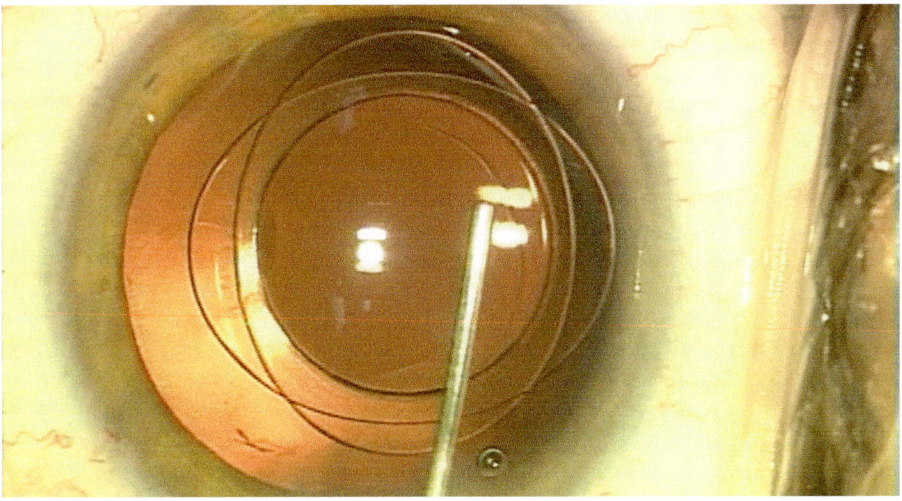

Fig. 11.2 Injection of Healon over the lens to push it back onto the capsule

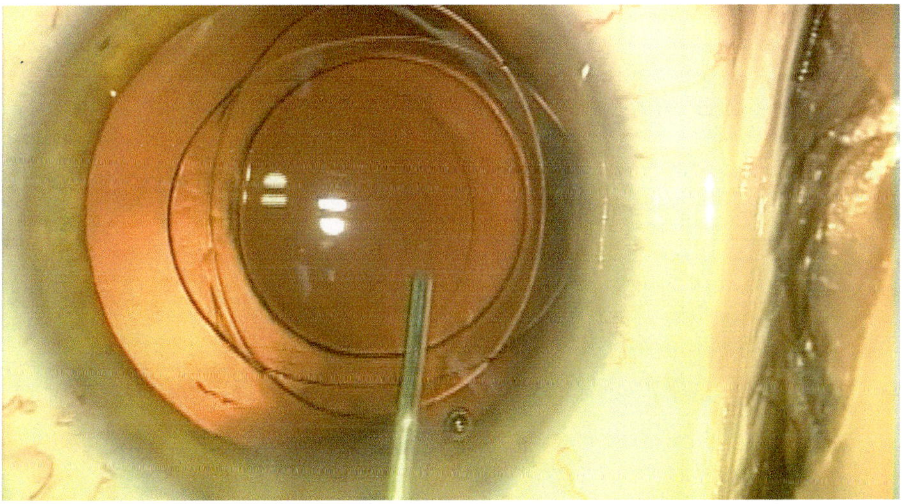

Fig. 11.3 Tilting the posterior haptic and catching both capsules in the lens groove

The lens implant is then gently moved vertically over and back from the surgeon's 12 o'clock position to encourage the capsules to slide into the lens groove, under the anterior haptics (Fig. 11.4). This process continues until the majority of the capsules are captured in the groove and only the second posterior haptic is still out of the capsule.

The OVD cannula is then used to gently push the second posterior haptic downwards (Fig. 11.5). Successful capsule capture is usually indicated by a "snapping"

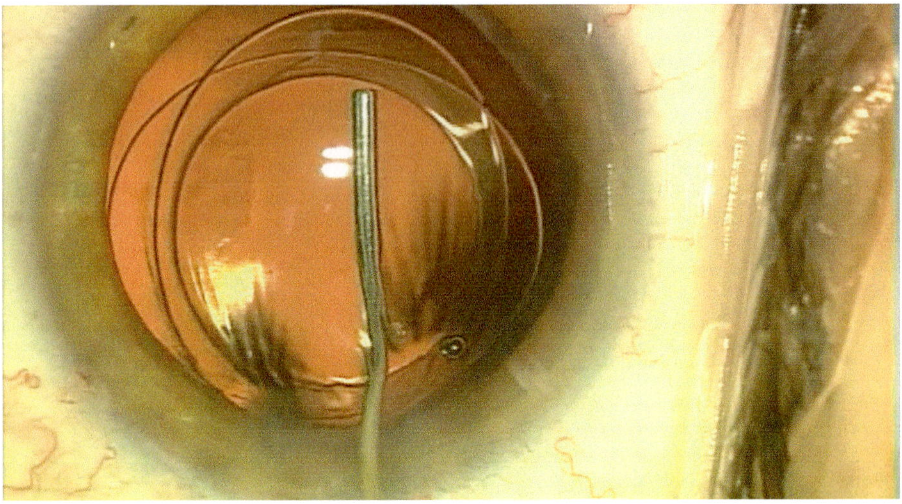

Fig. 11.4 Gentle vertical movements are used to encourage the capsules into the groove

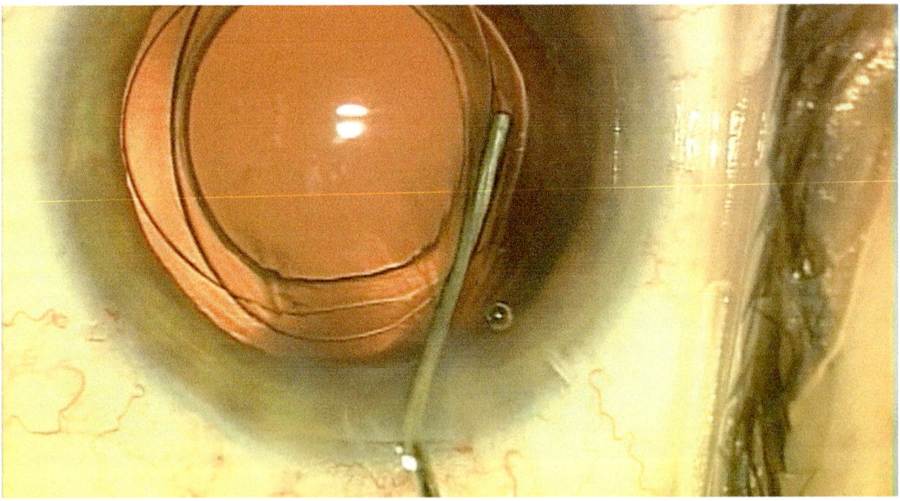

Fig. 11.5 Positioning the second posterior haptic and completing the insertion

of the rest of the capsule into the groove indicating correct lens positioning. During the learning curve, careful inspection of the lens and capsule at this point is needed to ensure that both capsules remain in the lens groove. During the learning curve, one of the challenges of the BIL technique involves keeping the anterior and posterior capsules together. This is key in making the lens implantation easier. This is achieved by counteracting the vitreous pressure and by maintaining a positive pressure in the anterior chamber.

11.4 Complications

Occasionally during injection, the BIL can partially prolapse through the capsular openings, into the space of Berger. The lens can also fall into the posterior segment in patients who have had a vitrectomy previously. This can be avoided by tilting the injector to keep the aperture angled in the direction of the anterior chamber or by using a side port instrument. This can be resolved easily if it does happen however. Using the OVD cannula, inject a cushion of OVD under the lens to lift it into the anterior chamber. This can position the lens where it needs to be for insertion without disturbing the anterior hyaloid face (Fig. 11.6).

An alternative implantation technique can be used, in the event that the capsular opening is a bit small or the zonulae are weak. The lens is first stabilized with the surgeon's non-dominant hand using a nucleus rotator. A hooked instrument is then slowly slid under the lens, and the capsular edge is grasped by the hook (Fig. 11.7). The lens is then held by one instrument, as the second instrument leads the bag gently into the groove. This technique is particularly useful when the lens is misbehaving and seems too tricky to insert in the normal way.

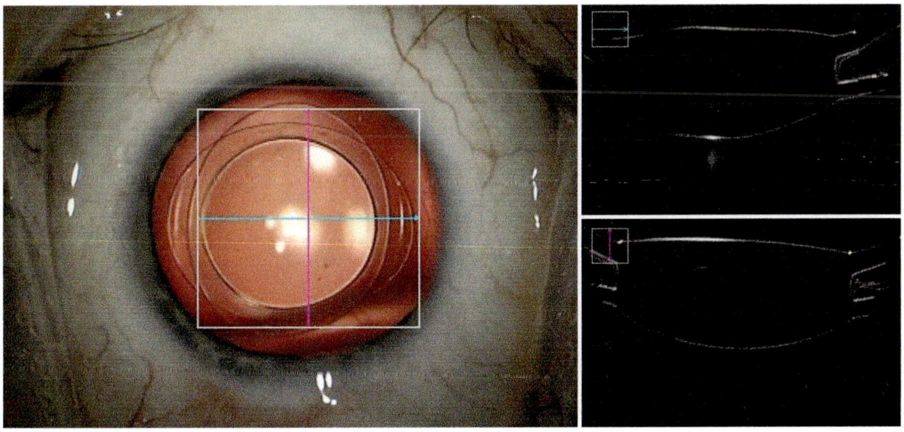

Time: 2015-03-05 10:36:05

Fig. 11.6 Intraoperative OCT imaging showing both capsular layers captured in the groove

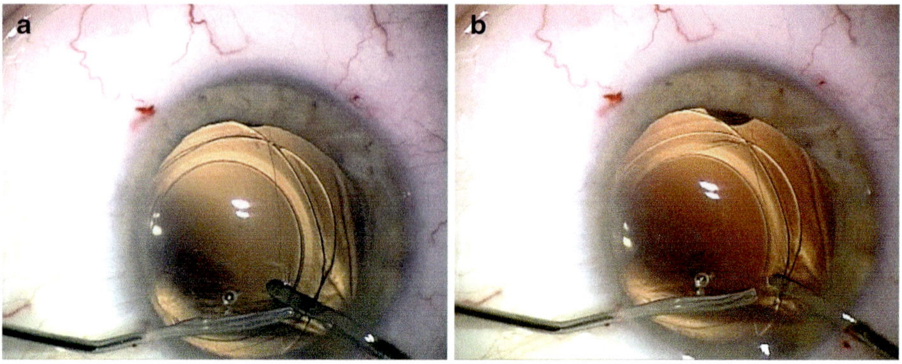

Fig. 11.7 Bimanual BIL implantation technique

11.5 Core Messages

- Ensure that the anterior and posterior capsules are apposed prior to lens insertion.
- If the capsules are not on top of each other, the IOL can be used to push the anterior capsule down to meet the posterior, bringing them together prior to inserting the IOL.
- If the anterior or posterior capsulorhexis is too small, enlarge the opening as described previously (Chap. 8).
- If there is any zonular weakness, the lack of countertraction can make insertion of the IOL very difficult; try using the bimanual insertion technique.

Toric BIL Implantation

12

Luc Van Os

12.1 Introduction

Cataract surgery offers the possibility to make a patient independent of spectacles. However, for a long time, corneal astigmatism was not corrected at the lenticular level when implanting an IOL during cataract surgery. With the introduction of toric intraocular lenses, the possibilities to improve uncorrected distance visual acuity (UCDVA) have become available. In a recent review, UCDVA was better, and there was more spectacle independence with toric IOLs than with non-toric IOLs [1].

As a consequence of its design, the centration of the BIL is very stable over time and can be accurately determined by the surgeon [2, 3]. Furthermore, the rotational stability of the BIL has proven to be very good, with a mean rotation of 0.36 ± 1.39° at 6 months after implantation [4]. It has also been proven that the surgically induced astigmatism (SIA) after BIL surgery with a 2.8 mm temporal self-sealing corneal incision is not statistically significant [5].

These three parameters indicate that the BIL is very suitable for adding a toric element to the IOL.

12.2 Indications for Toric BIL

It is important to differentiate the total astigmatism of the eye from the pure corneal astigmatism, which is the component that will be corrected when implanting a toric IOL. To that end, it is the keratometric values that are determinative to make the indication for a toric implant.

L. Van Os (✉)
Department of Ophthalmology, Antwerp University, University Hospital, Edegem, Belgium
e-mail: luc.vanos@uza.be

M.-J. Tassignon et al. (eds.), *Innovative Implantation Technique*,
https://doi.org/10.1007/978-3-030-03086-5_12

In a Danish series from 2002–2013, 20% of non-pediatric patients who underwent cataract surgery showed a preoperative corneal astigmatism of 1.5D or greater [6]. This indicates that the number of patients who might profit from a toric implant is quite important.

A toric BIL can be used for patients with corneal astigmatism of 1D or higher, as it has been proven that surgically induced astigmatism (SIA) is very low in BIL implantation with self-sealing temporal corneal incision [5]. In a study from our department, it was also shown that limited irregular astigmatism can also be corrected with a toric BIL, provided that the irregularity does not exceed 15° [7].

12.3 Pre-Surgical Planning and Calculation of the BIL

The toric element of the BIL is added on the anterior side of the optic, given that the optic power of the toric element is greater when it is closer to the cornea. The presence of the toric element on the anterior surface of the BIL is pointed out by two round etchings on the edge of the optic that indicate the cylinder axis.

The haptics of the toric BIL and the circumferential size of the lens are identical to the standard BIL design.

The formula used to calculate the IOL is based on the SRK/T formula but uses a customized A-constant approach [8].

For the calculation of the toric BIL, a customized worksheet functions as the order form for the implant. It includes the keratometric values and the axial length and proposes different IOL options with their respective planned outcome. Two schematic drawings are pictured, indicating the cylinder axis (bold black line), marked by the two etchings (represented by two red circles) and the power axis (yellow line). These can help as a final reminder of the correct lens position during surgery.

A new calculation sheet in which posterior corneal astigmatism is taken into account for the calculation of the implant has recently been developed and will be validated and compared to the existing formula in the near future.

For more detailed information on the calculation of the toric BIL, the paper written by Gobin et al. [8] is a valuable resource.

12.4 Surgical Technique

Before the actual surgery starts, axis markings are made on the corneal epithelium. Various techniques have been described to do this [9–11], which technique you use is not of importance in terms of the implantation of a toric BIL. You should use a technique that you feel comfortable or familiar with and that provides you with reliable and accurate marks.

Several microscope-assisted projections of the axis have recently become available or are in development. These can be very helpful for this part of the surgery in the future, but are not yet standard procedure in our hospital.

Once the surgery is initiated, special care should be taken regarding the centration of the ring caliper before performing the anterior capsulorhexis, as described in Chap. 6. Verifying the centration with the Eye Cage instrument is very helpful in these cases. It is also important not to oversize the capsulorhexis, as this might result in weaker constriction around the optic and thus in the possible rotation of the implant afterwards. The following steps of the surgery proceed as in a standard BIL surgery, again taking care for a carefully sized and matched posterior capsulorhexis.

When loading the IOL in the cartridge for injection, the toric element should be placed anteriorly; they can easily be recognized by the etchings that are added to indicate the cylinder axis. Loading the BIL under the microscope can offer additional reassurance of its correct positioning in the cartridge.

After the injection in the anterior chamber, it is helpful to already position the IOL according to the desired axis, before trapping the capsular blades in the peripheral groove. Rotating the IOL is easier while it is still unfixed in the anterior chamber, and it will avoid unnecessary traction on the capsular bag and zonular fibers. Once the IOL is approximately aligned in this way, the capsule is positioned in the groove as described in Chap. 9, and the last rotational movements toward the exact position can be performed. This is done by positioning a blunt instrument, such as the tip of the Rycroft cannula on the OVD syringe in the slight dip made by either of the two etchings on the lens surface. This offers enough grip to make small rotational movements. Once the lens is in the correct position, surgery can again proceed according to the usual protocol.

12.5 Complications

The main complications specific to toric BIL implantation are due to incorrect positioning of the BIL implant. It is important to remember that the etchings on the IOL indicate the cylinder axis, which will be perpendicular to the power axis. To avoid incorrect positioning, verify the positioning of the IOL by reviewing the patient's biometric parameters and the order form for the IOL before starting the surgery.

Another possible pitfall concerns positioning the IOL in the cartridge. The etchings on the IOL are on the same side as the toric element and should be anteriorly placed. Loading the lens under the microscope can be helpful in case you feel unsure about the position of the IOL in the cartridge. If the IOL is mistakenly implanted with the toric element positioned posteriorly, it can theoretically result in a decrease of up to 0.2 diopter in cylindrical power [8].

Postoperative rotation is rare but can occur. In this case, the rotation of the IOL can be done easily. Because the haptics do not go all the way into the capsular bag as is the case with more classic lens designs, it is easier to mobilize the lens within the rhexis ring. After mobilizing the lens, it can be rotated using a blunt instrument and taking hold of one of the etchings on the lens. If rotation reoccurs, for example, in cases where very little capsule fibrosis occurs, the placement of bean-shaped segments can help in stabilizing lens position (Chap. 18).

In cases with irregular astigmatism, a certain amount of astigmatism can persist. This can be addressed with the use of contact lenses or corneal refractive procedures.

12.6 Practical Example

A 44-year-old patient presented with a cataract related to myotonic dystrophy (Steinert disease). Preoperative biometric measures for the left eye are shown below (Figs. 12.1 and 12.2).

The keratometric data from the Scheimpflug imaging and the axial length from the biometry are then added to the order form, which exists as an Excel worksheet (imaged below: Fig. 12.3). The worksheet will generate different options with their respective expected outcomes. The surgeon can then adjust the suggested IOL to his or her liking and can then send the form to the manufacturer. Figure 12.4 shows the postoperative positioning of the IOL in this patient.

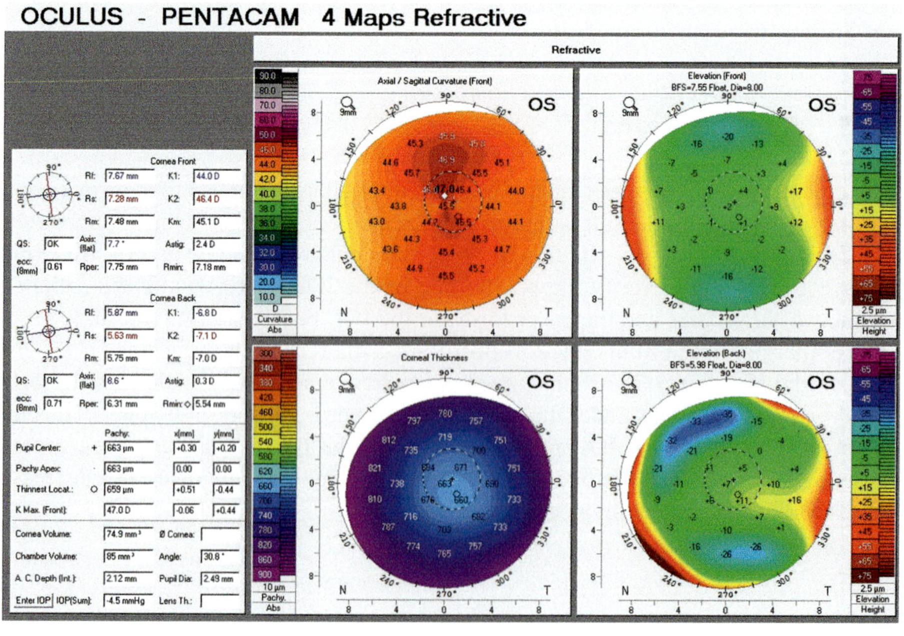

Fig. 12.1 Scheimpflug imaging of the left eye

Examination 1 of 6/08/14
Analysis 8, standardized
Biometry

Time: 14:42
Duration: 2 Min

		OD Right eye	OS Left eye
Measuring mode	Mode	Phakic	Phakic
Axial length	AL	⚠ 22,10 mm	22,15 mm
Cornea thickness	CCT	651 µm	662 µm
Aqueous depth	AD	2,20 mm	2,11 mm
Lens thickness	LT	5,03 mm	5,10 mm
Retina thickness	RT	200** µm	200** µm
Flat meridian	K1	44,29 D @ 175°	44,19 D @ 7°
Steep meridian	K2	47,17 D @ 85°	46,77 D @ 97°
Astigmatism	AST	2,88 D @ 85°	2,58 D @ 97°
Keratometric index	n	1,3375	1,3375
White to White	WTW	11,31 mm	11,42 mm
Iris barycenter	IC	-0,51 / -0,08 mm	0,53 / -0,07 mm
Pupil diameter	PD	4,22 mm	3,55 mm
Pupil barycenter	PC	-0,52 / 0,01 mm	0,47 / 0,09 mm

* Value user-defined
** System constant
⊕ Significant difference between OD and OS
⚠ see detail printout
n Analysis

LENSTAR LS 900® — EyeSuite™ Biometry, V2.0.1 — LS 900, SN 871, V 1.1.0 — HAAG-STREIT DIAGNOSTICS

Fig. 12.2 Haag-Streit Lenstar biometry

MORCHER® Implants
Ophthalmic innovations since 1955

To be sent to:
sales01@morcher.com

In case you still have questions before sending the order, please contact:
marie-jose.tassignon@uza.be

Surgeon: ____________ Patient ID: ____________

e-mail address: ____________ Order day: ____________

The biometrical values of the eye need to be completed with a comma, not a period !

A Constant Spherical part: 118,0

Anterior Positioning = 118.0 (Acoustic biometry)
Posterior Positioning = 119.0 (Acoustic biometry)

Variable A-constant for the toric element.

	OD				OS			
	K1 (flat)	Axis	K2 (steep)	Axis	K1 (flat)	Axis	K2 (steep)	Axis
K (D)					44,00	8	46,40	98
L (mm)					22,15			
Spherical equivalent of targeted refraction (D)	0				0			

	OD IOL power (D)	OD Refraction (D)	OS IOL power (D)		OS Refraction (D)	
IOL power -1.5			20	+2,5@ 8	0,77	-0,01@ 98
IOL power -1.0			20,5	+2,5@ 8	0,47	-0,03@ 98
IOL power -0.5			21	+2,5@ 8	0,16	-0,05@ 98
PROPOSAL IOL POWER			21,5	+2,5@ 8	-0,15	-0,07@ 98
IOL power +0.5			22	+2,5@ 8	-0,46	-0,09@ 98
IOL power +1.0			22,5	+2,5@ 8	-0,77	-0,11@ 98
IOL power +1.5			23	+2,5@ 8	-1,08	-0,13@ 98

Surgeon choice (if different from proposal)			@		21,5	2,0	@	10

Implantation axis. Please check for the edges of the toric element in the BIL is anteriorly positioned in the cartridge.

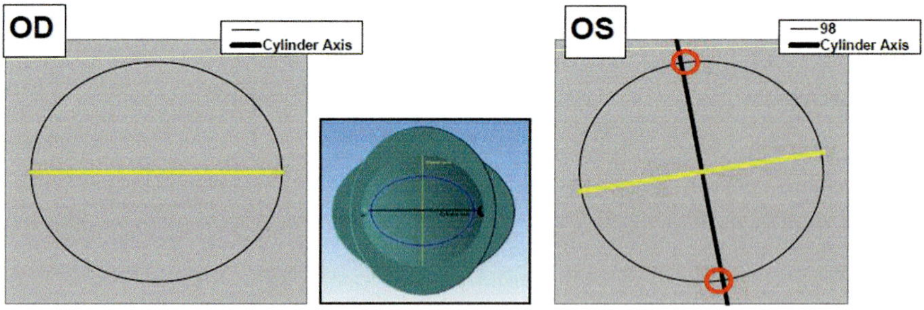

Fig. 12.3 Order form

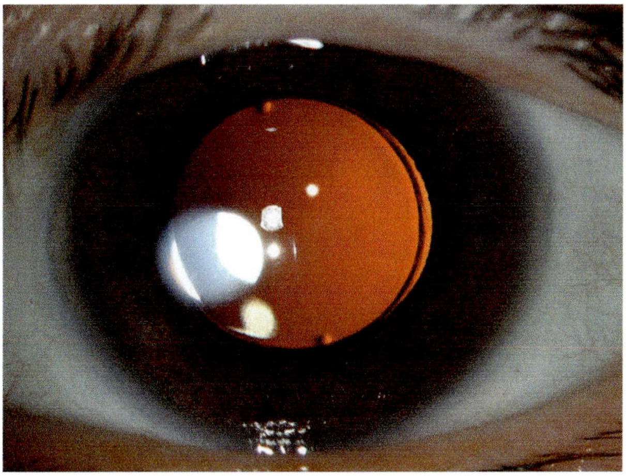

Fig. 12.4 Postoperative result (1 week after surgery) with the cylinder axis indication visible after pupil dilation

12.7 Core Messages

- BIL offers excellent and surgeon-controlled centration.
- BIL is rotationally stable.
- The round etchings on the lens indicate the cylinder axis.
- Toric element should be placed on the anterior side.

12.8 Instruments Used

The instruments listed are our preference but similar can be used based on the preference of the surgeon.

Item	Description	Manufacturer
OVD	Healon, Healon GV	Abbott Medical Optics, USA
Rycroft	OVD cannula	Steriseal, included in OVD package
Eye Cage	Alignment device	EyeTech LCD305B, UK
Bean-shaped segments (type 80 A–F)	Sulcus-positioned IOL-stabilizing device	Morcher, Germany

References

1. Kessel L, Andresen J, Tendal B, Erngaard D, Flesner P, Hjortdal J. Toric intraocular lenses in the correction of astigmatism during cataract surgery. Ophthalmology. 2016;113:275 86.
2. Verbruggen KHM, Rozema JJ, Gobin L, Coeckelbergh T, De Groot V, Tassignon M-J. Intraocular lens centration and visual outcomes after bag-in-the-lens implantation. J Cataract Refract Surg. 2007;33:1267–72.
3. Tassignon M-J, Rozema JJ, Gobin L. Ring-shaped caliper for better anterior capsulorhexis sizing and centration. J Cataract Refract Surg. 2006;32:1253–5.

4. Rozema JJ, Gobin L, Verbruggen K, Tassignon M-J. Changes in rotation after implantation of a bag-in-the-lens intraocular lens. J Cataract Refract Surg. 2009;35:1385–8.
5. Gobin L, Tassignon M-J, Wouters K, De Groot V. Surgically induced astigmatism after intraocular lens implantation using the bag-in-the-lens technique. J Cataract Refract Surg. 2011;37:1015–9.
6. Ostri C, Falck L, Boberg-Ans G, Kessel L. The need for toric intra-ocular lens implantation in public ophthalmology departments. Acta Ophthalmol. 2015;93:e396–7.
7. Tassignon M-J, Gobin L, Mathysen D, Van Looveren J. Clinical results after spherotoric intraocular lens implantation using the bag-in-the-lens technique. J Cataract Refract Surg. 2011;37:830–4.
8. Gobin L, Tassignon M-J, Mathysen D. Spherotoric bag-in-the-lens intraocular lens: power calculation and predictive misalignment nomogram. J Cataract Refract Surg. 2011;37:1020–30.
9. Visser N, Berendschot TTJM, Bauer NJC, Jurich J, Kersting O, Nuijts RMMA. Accuracy of toric intraocular lens implantation in cataract and refractive surgery. J Cataract Refract Surg. 2011;37:1394–402.
10. Onishi H, Torii H, Watanabe K, Tsubote K, Negishi K. Comparison of clinical outcomes among 3 marking methods for toric intraocular lens implantation. Jpn J Ophthalmol. 2016;60:142–9.
11. Farooqui JH, Koul A, Dutta R, Shroff NM. Comparison of two different methods of preoperative marking for toric intraocular lens implantation: bubble marker versus pendulum marker. Int J Ophthalmol. 2016;9:703–6.

The BIL Exchange Technique

13

Sorcha Ní Dhubhghaill and Clare Quigley

13.1 Introduction

Intraocular lenses are not typically implanted with the intention of removing them. Once a lens in the bag IOL is implanted within the capsule, a capsular response begins, mediated by the residual lens capsule epithelial cells (LECs) [1]. The cells proliferate and wrap around the optics and haptics of the implant. If such a lens needs to be explanted, separating the capsule from the implant can be extremely challenging, particularly in the regions around the haptics [2]. Lens design, biomaterial, duration of time in situ, and the presence of an Nd-Yag laser capsulotomy all influence the technical difficulty of removing an intraocular lens. Postoperative complications of lens in the bag IOL exchange may include posterior capsular opacification, vitreous prolapse, cystoid macular oedema, and increased astigmatism [3].

In the case of the BIL, the implant's unique design features haptics which rest outside of the capsule, sealing the LECs in the groove. This allows for the restriction of the LECs from encapsulating the lens as well as the well-recognised prevention of posterior capsular opacification. This results in an IOL that is significantly easier to remove and to replace than a lens in the bag, even many years after the original implantation.

S. Ní Dhubhghaill (✉)
Department of Ophthalmology, Antwerp University, University Hospital, Edegem, Belgium
e-mail: sorcha.nidhubhghaill@uza.be

C. Quigley
Department of Ophthalmology, Mater Misericordiae University Hospital, Dublin, Ireland

M.-J. Tassignon et al. (eds.), *Innovative Implantation Technique*,
https://doi.org/10.1007/978-3-030-03086-5_13

13.2 Indications for a BIL Exchange

Like most other hydrophilic acrylic intraocular lenses, the BIL is susceptible to optic opacification, though this occurs rarely [4]. In these cases, the opacification is due to the deposition of calcium and phosphorous within the IOL biomaterial. In the case that we reported, these opacities manifested clinically 10 years after the original implantation. We have estimated the rate of BIL opacification to be approximately 0.06% [4]. The other leading indication for BIL exchange in our centre is unexpected refractive outcome or 'refractive surprise'. It can occur in situations in which the preoperative measurements, on the basis of which the IOL power is calculated, are not sufficiently accurate. This tends to occur in 'outlier' cases such as extreme myopia and hypermetropia, previous radial keratotomy (RK) and keratoconus in our centre. An increasing indication is also provided by the dissatisfied minority of patients who receive multifocal IOLs (MIOLs) and experience vision quality problems including glare and blur.

13.3 Surgical Technique

Surgery may be performed under topical or regional anaesthesia, based on the surgeon's preference. We recommend a 3-step temporal main incision of 2.8 mm and a 1 mm paracentesis. An intracameral injection of 0.1 mL adrenaline (1:1000) diluted in 0.9 mL preservative-free xylocaine is used to supplement the anaesthesia and pupil dilation. Ophthalmic viscosurgical device (OVD) is then injected into the anterior chamber. Our preferred OVD for this purpose is Healon GV (Abbott Medical Optics, USA). The lens can then be mobilised and released from the capsular bag by rotating the IOL. If the implant can be rotated, the capsule is free and unstuck, thereby making the subsequent step easier. An IOL rotator (Bausch & Lomb) and the OVD cannula are used to disengage the bag from the groove of the BIL (Fig. 13.1).

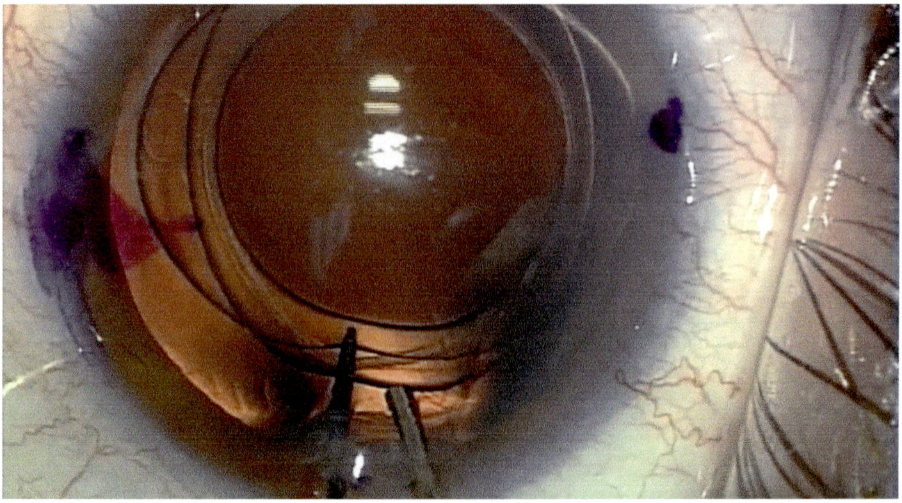

Fig. 13.1 Disengaging the lens from the capsule

Once a little gap has been made, the OVD cannula can be advanced behind the lens and a cushion of OVD can be injected behind the lens optic (Fig. 13.2).

This has the combined benefits of both pushing the lens up into the anterior chamber and also pushing the anterior hyaloid down, thereby preventing vitreous prolapse during the removal. We use a lasso lens cutter (Moria Surgical, France) to bisect the lens, though a Vannas scissors or a femtosecond laser may also be used [4]. The lasso is inserted into the anterior chamber through the main incision and by a microforceps in the paracentesis. Using the forceps, the edge of the lens can be grasped and threaded through the loop of the cutter (Fig. 13.3).

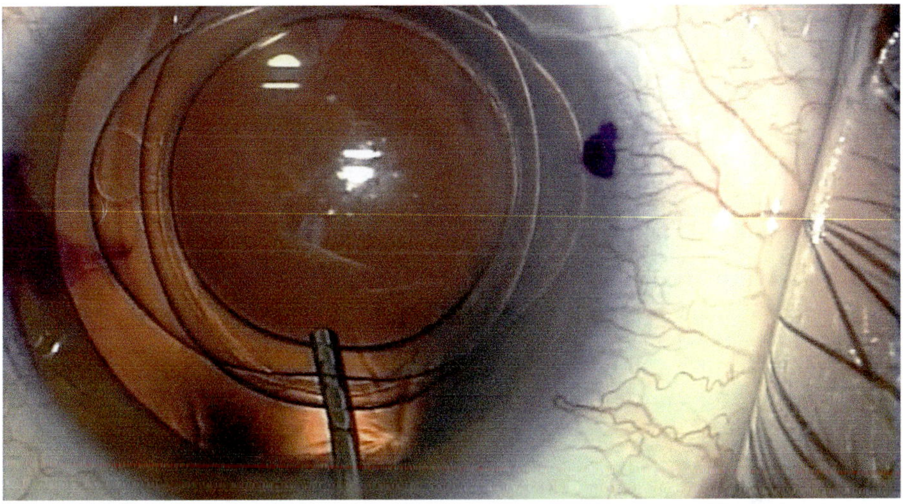

Fig. 13.2 Injecting OVD behind the lens to lift it into the anterior chamber

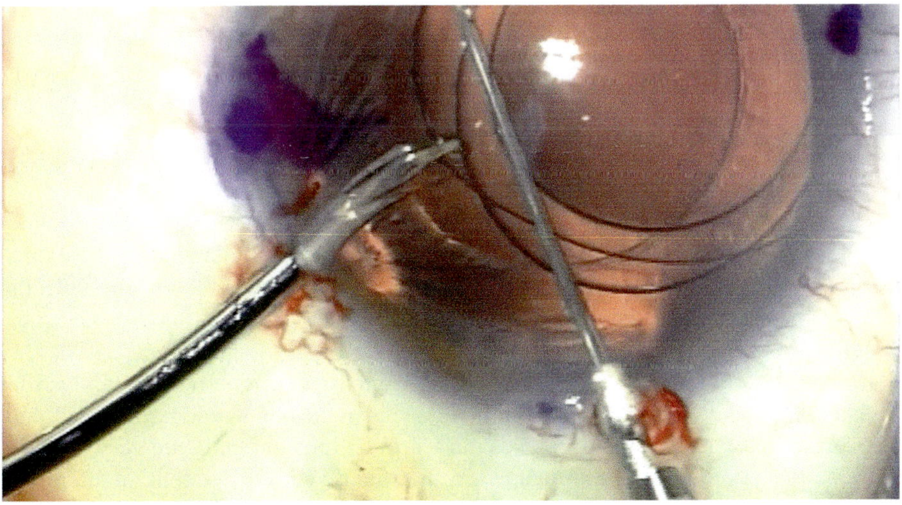

Fig. 13.3 Guiding the lens into the lasso with the microforceps

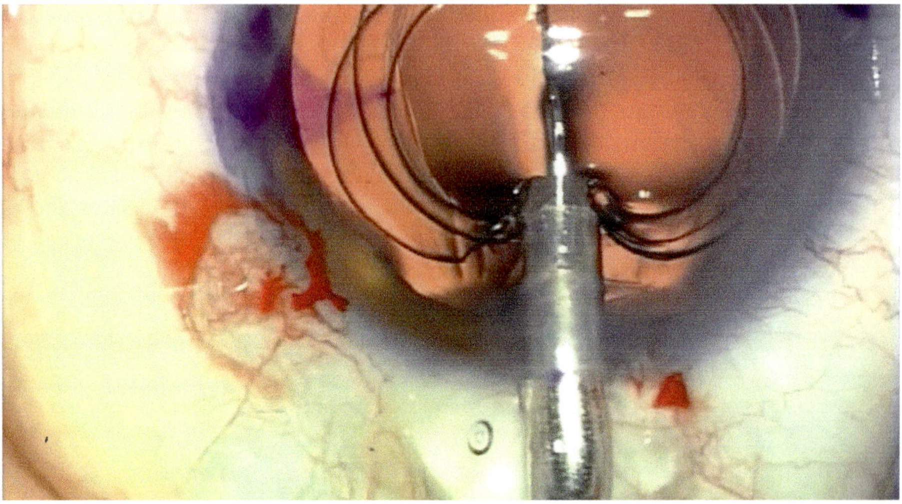

Fig. 13.4 The slow squeezing mechanism of the loop will bisect the lens in a controlled way

The lens is advanced until it is aligned in the centre of the loop, with the haptics adopting an X shape. The microforceps can then be removed to allow for the two-handed cutting movement to bisect the lens. The lasso can be used to cut lenses up to +30 dioptres, though thicker lenses take more effort to cut and should be done slowly (Fig. 13.4).

A toothed forceps can be used to remove the two lens pieces. If the lens pieces are still too difficult to remove, then the wound can be enlarged or the lasso can be used to cut the lens even smaller. When all the lens pieces have been removed, the anterior chamber should be inspected to ensure that there is no presence of vitreous prolapse. In most cases the cushion of OVD is enough to tamponade the vitreous, but if the lens removal is difficult, then an anterior vitrectomy may be required. Once this step has been completed, a new BIL can be injected into the anterior chamber and implanted into the opening in the same way as with the original lens. The case can then be completed like a normal BIL procedure as described previously.

13.4 Complications

The lens pieces should be grasped by the optic, rather than by the haptic, given that they tend to break during extraction. Scissors can also be used to cut the IOL, but great care should be taken to keep the lens stable and to prevent disturbance to the anterior hyaloid. It should also be noted that the best lens to replace a BIL is another BIL. The anterior and posterior capsules begin to fuse relatively quickly after implantation, and opening them to implant a lens in the bag would be very difficult. The presence of a PPCCC also makes intracapsular lens implantation very difficult. A three-piece lens could be implanted in the sulcus, with or without an attempt at optic capture, but we would still advise a BIL wherever possible.

13.5 Core Messages

- Rotate the BIL before trying to remove it to ensure the capsule is completely unstuck.
- Disengage the lens at the surgeon's 12 o'clock position by retrieving the capsules out of the lens groove and pushing the posterior haptic down towards the vitreous allowing to Healon needle to find its way behind the lens optic.
- Inject a cushion of OVD behind the lens optic to lift the lens out of the capsule, into the anterior chamber.
- A lens lasso provides a very controlled way to bisect the IOL in situ and can work for lenses up to +30 dioptres.

13.6 Instruments Used

The instruments listed are our preference, but similar ones can be used based according to the surgeon's preference.

Item	Description	Manufacturer
OVD	Healon, Healon GV	Abbott Medical Optics, USA
IOL rotator	Spatula	Bausch & Lomb
Rycroft	OVD cannula	Steriseal, included in OVD package
Microforceps	Ikeda angled 30° Capsulorhexis 23.0 g forceps	EyeTech Fr2268
IOL lasso cutter	Looped wire IOL lens cutter	Moria Surgical Instruments, France

References

1. Joo C-KSJ-A, Kim J-H. Capsular opening contraction after continuous curvilinear capsulorhexis and intraocular lens implantation. J Cataract Refract Surg. 1996;22:585–90.
2. Leysen I, Bartholomeeusen E, Coeckelbergh T, Tassignon MJ. Surgical outcomes of intraocular lens exchange: five year study. J Cataract Refract Surg. 2009;35:1013–8.
3. Ni Dhubhghaill S, Van Os L, De Keizer RJW, Taal M, Zakaria N, Tassignon MJ. Intraocular lens exchange technique for an opacified bag-in-the-lens. J Cataract Refract Surg. 2015;41:924–8.
4. Bala CPU, Chan T, Shi J, Meades K. Transection and explantation of intraocular lenses using femtosecond lasers. J Cataract Refract Surg. 2017;43:420–3.

Femtosecond Bag-in-the-Lens Cataract Surgery

14

H. Burkhard Dick, Tim Schultz, and Ronald D. Gerste

14.1 Introduction

That phacoemulsification is the leading, maybe even the optimal, method to perform cataract surgery is a notion that is widely shared by many ophthalmologists. But as if giving life to the old conventional wisdom that good is good but better carries it, an increasing number of cataract surgeons have embraced a new technology introduced by Zoltan Z Nagy in 2008. The femtosecond laser was already well established in corneal refractive surgery; its use in cataract surgery has grown steadily over the last decade. The femtosecond laser can – as of now – perform corneal incisions, capsulotomy, lens fragmentation, and arcuate incisions to treat astigmatism.

Whether femtosecond laser-assisted cataract surgery (usually abbreviated as LCS = laser cataract surgery) is actually better than conventional phacoemulsification or what the distinct advantages of the one method over the others are has been the subject of a number of studies and published personal opinions. The final verdict has not yet been spoken and probably never will – laser cataract surgery is an ongoing development, and current techniques might be improved if not outdated within just a few years.

Some studies trying to assess the merits of one method versus the other suffer, however, from lack of an adequate matching. Comparing phacoemulsification

H. Burkhard Dick · R. D. Gerste
University Eye Hospital, Bochum, North-Rhine Westphalia, Germany
e-mail: burkhard.dick@kk-bochum.de

T. Schultz (✉)
Ophthalmologist, Historian, Washington, DC, USA
e-mail: Tim.Schultz@kk-bochum.de

M.-J. Tassignon et al. (eds.), *Innovative Implantation Technique*,
https://doi.org/10.1007/978-3-030-03086-5_14

versus LCS sometimes resembles the old adage of apples that cannot be compared to oranges. Patients choosing LCS to a large degree opt for a premium IOL. One large, recent study compared more than 2800 LCS cases with almost 5000 conventional phacoemulsification cases. In the former group, multifocal, toric, multifocal toric, and accommodating IOLs were inserted in almost 43% of the LCS group – and in a combined less than 1% in the standard phacoemulsification group. The limits of comparing two populations with such huge differences are quite obvious [1].

A Cochrane review based on 16 randomized controlled trials (RCTs) enrolling a total of 1638 eyes found little evidence of any important difference in postoperative visual acuity between LCS and standard phacoemulsification; a small advantage for LCS was noted at 6 months in best-corrected distance visual acuity (CDVA) [2]. A recent analysis based on 14,567 eyes from 15 randomized trials and 22 observational studies found no statistically significant differences between the two methods in postoperative corrected as well as uncorrected distance visual acuity and in postoperative refractive error. Some safety parameters were significantly in favor of LCS like capsulotomy circularity, postoperative corneal thickness, and in the reduction of corneal endothelial cells [3, 4]. In most of our patients, we are able to perform cataract extraction and IOL implantation with "zero phaco" – without any ultrasound utilization at all. That, in our view, contributes to the high safety profile of LCS.

The femtosecond laser has proven particularly precise and effective when it comes to opening the capsule. It has been well established that the femtosecond laser creates better capsulotomy geometry and circularity than the manual capsulorhexis [5]. Numerous studies confirmed that these circular capsular openings surpass the manual technique of continuous curvilinear capsulorhexis with improved IOL-capsule overlap. Capsulotomies performed by the femtosecond laser reduce the probability of IOL decentration and tilt [6]. The earlier the capsular bag diameter stabilizes, the better for a more predictable effective lens position, IOL power calculations, and refractive outcomes. Measuring capsular bag shrinkage in 53 eyes that underwent LCS and in 53 fellow eyes that underwent manual phacoemulsification, the LCS group had significantly less capsular bag shrinkage than the standard group at 1, 2, and 3 months, with a mean difference of 0.33 ± 0.25 mm at 3 months [7].

The impressive precision of the laser pretreatment and its safety are factors of significance when planning surgery with a sophisticated approach – like bag-in-the-lens.

14.2 Methods/Technique

As other authors in this volume have well noted, creating appropriately sized and centered capsulorhexes relative to each other is important in BIL implantation. An optimal IOL centration is dependent on the position of the two capsulorhexes [8], the latter being a term used for manually performed continuous curvilinear capsulorhexis (CCC), while the same step performed by a laser system should more adequately be called a capsulotomy [9]. In BIL implantation, creating a manual posterior capsulorhexis has repeatedly been described as being quite demanding, maybe even impossible in some cases [10].

The femtosecond laser with its ability to create perfectly centered, reproducible circular capsule openings can be employed for both anterior and posterior capsulotomies. In our experience, facilitating the creation of the posterior capsulotomy with an image-guided femtosecond laser provides precise control of size and centration symmetry with the anterior capsulotomy and reproducibility that is technically difficult with traditional manual techniques.

The surgical technique of employing the femtosecond laser in BIL cataract surgery can be described in ten steps.

14.2.1 Step 1: Planning

While in LCS the patient is normally docked to the laser (we are using the Catalys platform [Johnson and Johnson Vision]) and the different steps – anterior capsulotomy, lens fragmentation, and corneal incisions, if desired – are done in short succession, femtosecond BIL cataract surgery requires two separate laser treatments for each eye. The treatment parameters we are usually choosing are 5.0 mm diameter and pulse energy of 4 mJ for the anterior capsulotomy. The incision depth is 600 mm. For the lens fragmentation, grid spacing of 350 mm or 500 mm and pulse energy of 9.5–10 mJ are used. For the second capsulotomy treatment, a 4.6 mm diameter posterior capsulotomy with energy of 4 to 10 μJ is used (Fig. 14.1).

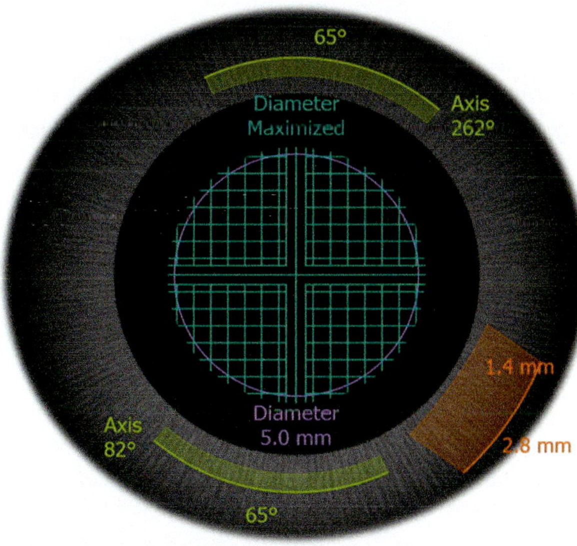

Fig. 14.1 Laser planning screen with corneal main incision, arcuate incisions, capsulotomy, and lens fragmentation

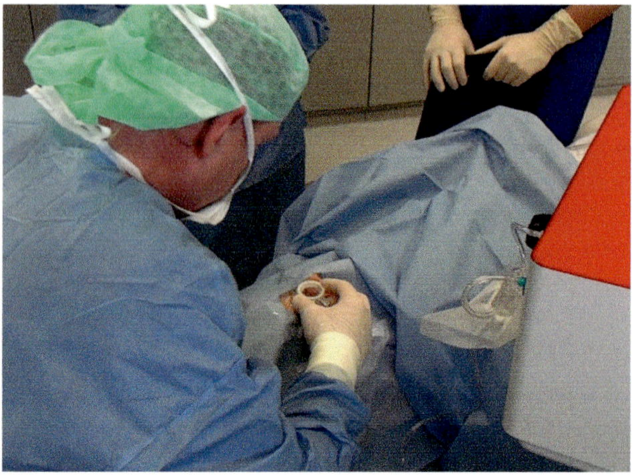

Fig. 14.2 Sterile positioning of the suction ring on the eye of the patient

14.2.2 Step 2: First Docking

The suction ring (Liquid Optics interface [Johnson and Johnson Vision]) is placed on the eye, and the first vacuum is activated to stabilize the eye. The suction ring is then filled with a balanced salt solution. A second suction is created between the suction ring and the non-applanating disposable lens (Fig. 14.2).

14.2.3 Step 3: Image Guidance

The three-dimensional full-volume optical coherence tomography (SD-OCT) image guidance system will determine the location and dimension of the cornea, the anterior chamber, the anterior capsule, and the posterior capsule, as well as the thickness of the crystalline lens. In almost all cases, the software automatically identifies the surfaces, and the surgeon has to confirm only the planned treatment that was customized based on the anatomical surfaces of the eye. The anterior capsulotomy can be centered automatically on the pupil or the scanned capsule. Additionally, the high-resolution cross sections of the anterior segment displayed to the surgeon often provide visualization of Berger's space and the anterior hyaloid surface, knowledge of which can be valuable in subsequent steps in the technique (Fig. 14.3).

14.2.4 Step 4: Laser Treatment

The surgeon confirms the treatment plan and presses the pedal to commence treatment. On this first docking, the anterior capsulotomy, lens fragmentation (segmentation and softening), and corneal incisions (if desired) are performed. After finishing the laser treatment, the surgeon undocks the eye and proceeds with lens

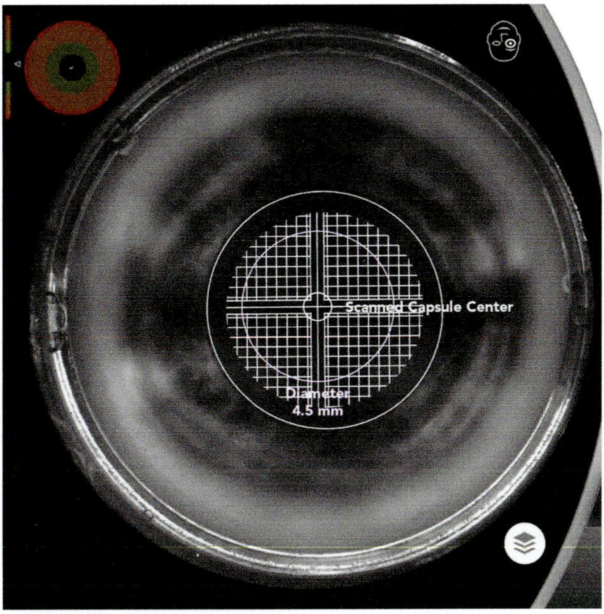

Fig. 14.3 Infrared camera view of the laser system. The capsulotomy is centered on the capsular bag, the fragmentation of lens on the pupil

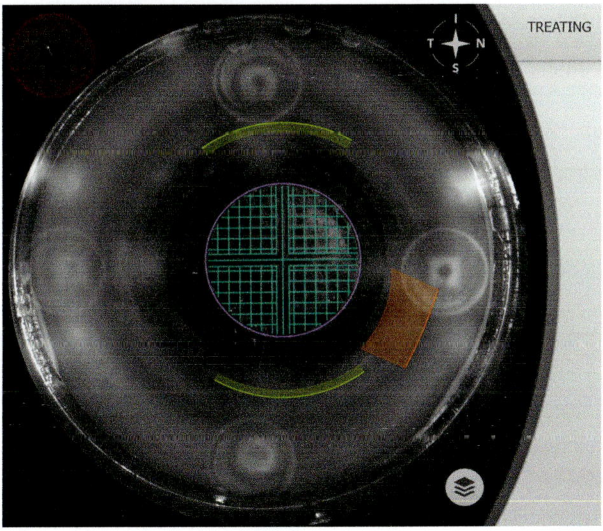

Fig. 14.4 Infrared camera view of the laser system during the treatment in a case with arcuate incisions and corneal main incision

removal. After the initial laser treatment, the patient interface is stored in a sterile cup holder (Fig. 14.4).

14.2.5 Step 5: Phacoemulsification and Lens Removal

The lens is removed like in any routine cataract surgery; using irrigation/aspiration in softened cataracts and phacoemulsification in denser, harder lenses (Fig. 14.5).

14.2.6 Step 6: Preparation for the Creation of the Posterior Capsulotomy

After the cortex is aspirated, the posterior capsule is carefully opened with a 27-gauge self-bent needle. Sodium hyaluronate 1% (Healon) is injected posteriorly to push back the intact anterior vitreous surface and elevate the posterior capsule. An ophthalmic viscosurgical device (OVD) is also injected into the anterior chamber to reform it. The incisions are hydrated with balanced salt solution. No sutures are necessary in adults (Fig. 14.6).

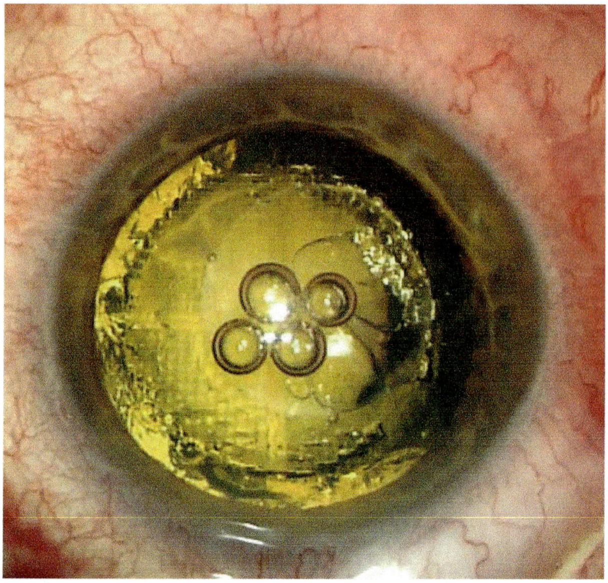

Fig. 14.5 Dens nucleus directly after laser treatment prior to manual removal

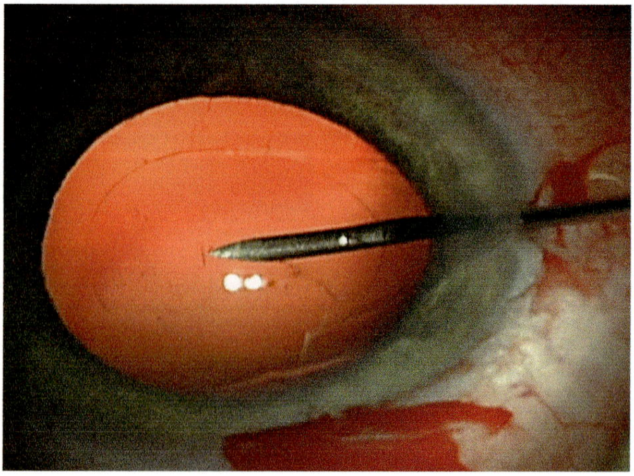

Fig. 14.6 Puncturing of the posterior capsule

14.2.7 Step 7: Second Docking

The patient is swiveled back to the femtosecond cataract laser. He or she is docked again for the posterior capsulotomy.

14.2.8 Step 8: Image Guidance

The OCT image guidance system will scan the eye, process the full-volume data, and attempt to identify the anatomical surfaces of the eye. At this time, the system will advise that modifications are required because abnormal anatomy has been detected. The surgeon is instructed by the system to confirm and adjust the surface fits for the anterior and posterior lens. In this specific situation, this message should be ignored. The high-resolution axial and sagittal OCT images will show the less than 5 μm thick posterior capsule in a convex shape, the anterior hyaloid in a concave shape, and a space between them, which was filled with OVD. The surfaces, from which the safety zones and the treatment are calculated, have to be customized. The convex surface in the anterior image (the posterior capsule) is customized and interpreted as the anterior capsule, the concave surface in the posterior image (the anterior hyaloid) is customized and interpreted as the posterior capsule, and the space between them is interpreted as the lens. Because the capsulotomy treatment is calculated based on what the user confirms as the correct surface, the planned capsulotomy can be delivered to the posterior capsule to create a posterior capsulotomy. The infrared camera picture is used to center the posterior capsulotomy to the anterior capsulotomy, and the intended location of the posterior capsulotomy is checked to be within the diameter of the anterior capsulotomy, usually with a 4.5–4.8 mm diameter (Fig. 14.7).

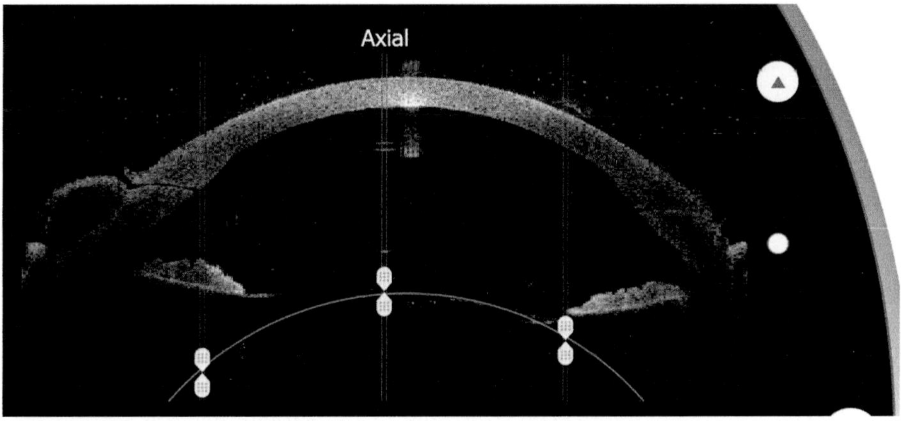

Fig. 14.7 Positioning of the treatment zone of the anterior capsulotomy on the posterior capsulotomy

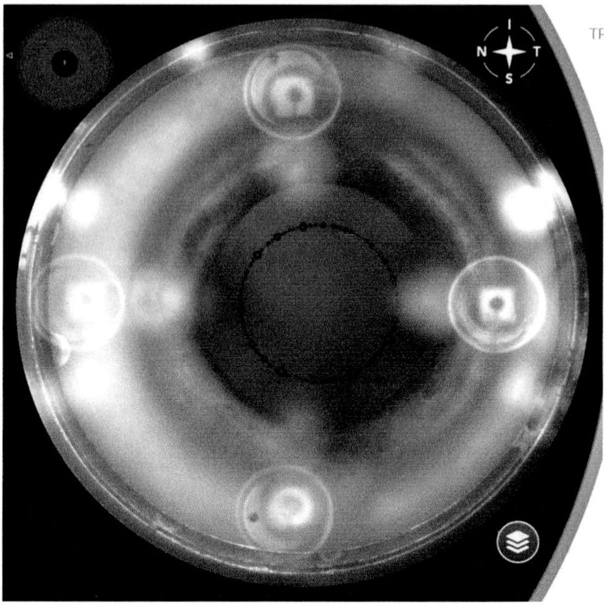

Fig. 14.8 During the posterior laser capsulotomy small bubbles can be seen

14.2.9 Step 9: Laser Treatment

In this step, the main asset of the femtosecond laser in BIL cataract surgery becomes evident: primary posterior capsulotomy is basically always possible and does not require any manual skills. The laser treatment time for the posterior capsulotomy is usually 12–14 s (Fig. 14.8).

14.2.10 Step 10: Implantation of the BIL

After the vacuum is released and the patient undocked, the patient is rotated back under the operating microscope. The edges of the posterior capsulotomy are easily seen due to the created gas bubbles. The anterior chamber is filled with sodium hyaluronate 1%. Using a microforceps, the surgeon verifies that the posterior capsulotomy was completed and carefully removes it. The main incision is then enlarged to 2.8 mm. The BIL type 89 A (Morcher GmbH), a foldable hydrophilic one-piece IOL we are using, is loaded into a 2.8 cartridge (Medicel) and injected into the anterior chamber. At the time of the injection, a spatula is placed beneath the IOL to prevent its injection into the vitreous. After the IOL is completely inserted and unfolded in the anterior chamber, the posterior haptics are placed behind the posterior capsule and the anterior haptics in front of the anterior capsule, keeping the anterior and posterior capsules in the IOL's flange. After IOL placement, the OVD is aspirated. Acetylcholine chloride is injected into the anterior chamber to bring the

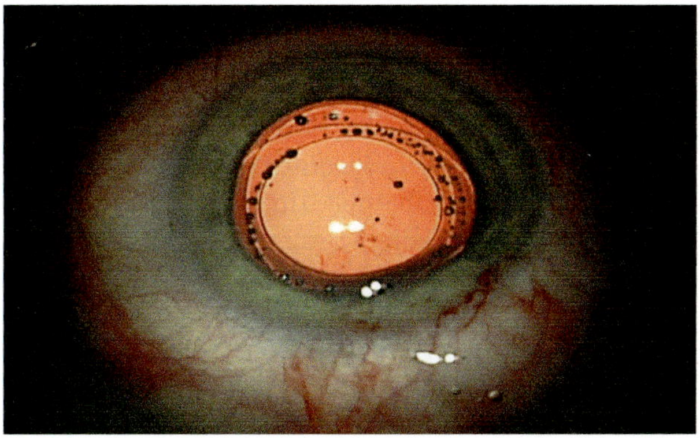

Fig. 14.9 Bag-in-the-lens after implantation

pupil to miosis. The paracentesis and main incision are closed watertight, if necessary by stromal hydration. At the end of surgery, one drop of pilocarpine 2% is instilled to maintain miosis (Fig. 14.9).

We have earlier published a series of 31 cases of femtosecond laser-assisted BIL, 6 men and 25 women with an average age of 73.5 years ±8.0 (SD) (range 59–91 years). There were no problems with intraocular pressure (IOP) during or after surgery, with the highest IOP measured postoperatively at 20 mm Hg. The corrected distance visual acuity (CDVA) (logMAR) was 0.44 ± 0.17 (range 0.2–1.0) preoperatively and 0.08 ± 0.11 (range 0.1–0.3) at 1 month. The CDVA increased in all patients postoperatively ($P < 0.0005$). Twenty-seven (87%) of the eyes were within 0.5 D of the target refraction at 1 month [11].

Femtosecond laser BIL cataract surgery in adult patients like these is impressive in several instances. The capsulotomy centration – and as a consequence the IOL centration – is excellent. The diameter of the capsulotomy can precisely be adjusted to the requirements of the specific IOL to be implanted. The position of the anterior capsule is well known as the final optic position of BIL IOLs. Any capsular bag shrinkage would not affect the IOL position in the postoperative period. As perfect as the centrations of the capsulotomy are its circularity we have not encountered any tension folds and the alignment of the posterior capsulotomy with the anterior capsulotomy. Since it is easily possible to preserve the anterior vitreous membrane, the formation of PCO is prevented. The stability of the IOL alignment that might not change at all over time makes BIL – manually, but in particular with the femtosecond laser – an ideal choice for sophisticated lenses like toric and multifocal IOLs.

14.3 Complications and Caveats

Postoperative care is not different from routine cataract surgery. In more than 90 patients operated so far, we did not encounter intraoperative or postoperative complications like fibrin reaction, cystoid macula edema, or other problems. Our experience, therefore, is not different from those of this book's editor/primary author: Marie-Jose Tassignon has reported a very low complication rate after manual BIL implantation in 807 eyes [10].

The surgeon has to be aware of a specific characteristic of femtosecond laser treatment: it increases the levels of prostaglandins in the aqueous humor, most likely due to mechanical or thermal stimuli. When we collected aqueous humor from 113 patients who during cataract surgery either had just undergone femtosecond laser treatment or – in the control group of 107 eyes – before commencing conventional phacoemulsification, the differences were indeed astonishing. In the femtosecond laser group, the average level of prostaglandin E_2 in one part of the study was 182 pg/ml – more than tenfold the concentration of PGE_2 in the control group, which was 17.3 pg/ml. This does not need, however, to cause alarm. Administering nonsteroidal anti-inflammatory drugs (NSAID), one eye drop three times on the day of surgery before initiating treatment, has reliably prevented intraoperative miosis (a consequence of elevated prostaglandin levels and highly unwelcome during cataract surgery) and seems to have reduced the risk of inflammation significantly [12].

There are certain system and logistical requirements for successful femtosecond laser BIL cataract surgery. Among the current imaging options, having a high-resolution 3D SD OCT is absolutely essential since only this device delivers the precision necessary, in particular for the posterior capsulotomy. For this step is so crucial in BIL cataract surgery, there is no regular applanation since the globe is still open at that time; the interface will be connected to the eye by posterior limbal docking.

The fact that in BIL cataract surgery – unlike in other LCS procedures – the laser is required for a second time after lens removal to perform the posterior capsulotomy makes it evident that the platform has to be positioned in the sterile environment of the operating room. In some institutions, there is a separation between a so-called laser suite and the operating room with the patient being pre-treated in the former and the surgery (mainly lens removal and IOL implantation) is performed in the latter. There are convincing reasons for the placement of the laser in the operating room beyond the specific necessities of BIL cataract surgery. One is avoiding a miotic eye on the operating table. If the pupil is smaller than the intended diameter of the laser-guided capsulotomy, the procedure will become difficult. Chances of encountering miosis are proverbially increasing with every minute gone by since laser treatment. The time-lapse caused by shuttling the patient from one room to another – maybe across a hallway – and then spending some time in a waiting room is a main cause for miosis, the reduction of pupil size mainly caused by the increased prostaglandin levels described above. There is a second argument for placing the laser in the operating room: separately used "laser suites" are usually described as "clean" – which from a hygienist's point of view means: unsterile. We have conducted histological studies on a human eye that was scheduled for enucleation after laser treatment. High-magnification light microscopy revealed complete cuts through several corneal layers with only minimal tissue bridges left in place. Therefore, after the corneal incision was made with the femtosecond laser, the eye must be considered "open" [13]. Therefore, a sterile environment and the use of sterile tools like the interfaces of which a second one should be employed for the posterior capsulotomy is indispensable.

Finally, there is an economical consideration. In most healthcare systems, the femtosecond laser application in BIL cataract surgery is regarded as two separate interventions resulting in "two-click fees" and thus rendering the operation too expensive. It is within the responsibility of the industry to come up with a solution – unfortunately, there is right now no specific software program adjusted to performing posterior capsulotomy.

14.4 Instruments

The one instrument we are using that is different from the tools described in the other chapters is the laser platform. The Catalys Precision Laser System, designed at that time by OptiMedica (Sunnyvale, CA) and until very recently distributed by Advanced Medical Optics (AMO) before being acquired by Johnson & Johnson (New Brunswick, New Jersey), has been introduced into clinical practice in Europe in 2011. Unlike other femtosecond systems in use in cataract surgery, Catalys does not have its origins in a device used for Lasik. The manufacturer designed the system exclusively with the lens (which requires a lower numerical aperture) in mind. Unique to the Catalys system are two features: the Liquid Optics interface docking system and an integrated spectral-domain optical coherence tomography (OCT) which is the core of the Catalys Integral Guidance system. The OCT is enhanced by sophisticated algorithms designed to ensure that the femtosecond laser pulses are delivered precisely to the intended location.

The system allows for a template-based planning approach with its touch screen graphic user interface. The surgeon can create a set of templates for anterior capsulotomy and lens fragmentation. Different treatment plans are stored in the laser system's database which allows the surgeon to choose a plan in advance of the procedure instead of entering the data after the patient is docked. Customized anterior capsulotomy and lens fragmentation patterns are overlaid onto the OCT data and projected onto the graphic user screen enabling the surgeon to adjust – if necessary – the position of the treatment zones depending on the anatomy and the position of the eye. The surgeon confirms the automated surface identification markers, safety margins, and treatment zones before commencing the laser application.

The Catalys systems introduced a new docking technology after various complications associated with existing interfaces like corneal damage, a significant rise in intraocular pressure, and difficulties with variations in orbital anatomy were reported. The Catalys' Liquid Optics interface includes a fluid-filled suction ring and a non-applanating disposable lens. The novel interface docks the patient to the system and is designed to provide a clear optical path for real-time video, OCT imaging, and laser treatment. Due to a rather gentle docking process, intraocular pressure rises only mildly, which is particularly important for older cataract patients, and minimizing scleral contact of the interface results in less redness of the eye after surgery.

In more than 99% of eyes operated with the Catalys system, free-floating capsulotomies in all corners were achieved. The capsulotomies were of a perfect diameter, position, shape, and centration and provided thus the best conditions for the implantation of premium IOL, like aspheric, multifocal, toric, and accommodating IOL [14].

This laser system has proven its reliability and safety in more than 9000 cataract operations in many if which the BIL technique has been used – in both – adult and pediatric patients with excellent results and high patient (or, in the latter case, parent) satisfaction.

14.5 Additional Headings: Femtosecond BIL Cataract Surgery in Children

There is one group of patients where the cataract surgeon's care takes on a completely new dimension: the youngest. Boys and girls with pediatric cataract, whether their lens opacification is congenital, infantile, or juvenile, whether they will undergo surgery at an age of 3 months, 3 years, or as a young (almost) adult at age 17, will bear the results of the cataract surgeon's endeavors for an entire lifetime which (given current life expectancies in the industrialized world) means probably for 70 and 80 years. It is thus of prime importance to provide these young patients with the best we can offer them – which in many cases means employing the femtosecond laser and also to implant a BIL.

Our experience with almost 9000 femtosecond laser-assisted cataract operations in adults convinced us that for many infants performing capsulotomy with the laser – one of the most crucial steps of the entire procedure – might be the right thing to do (as an off-label procedure, like so many surgical interventions in the infant eye). The manufacturer has introduced a smaller Liquid Optic interface especially for patients with tight palpebral fissures; this interface measures only 12 mm in diameter. The procedure of docking, scanning, and initiating the laser capsulotomy is very similar to what we do in elderly patients though some of the treatment data are a bit different. The incision depths vary from 400 to 1000 μm; pulse energy is set between 4 and 10 μJ. The intended diameter of the anterior capsulotomy is between 3.3 and 5.2 mm, for the posterior capsulotomy the diameter is between 3.2 and 4.7 mm.

It is safe, convenient, and timesaving to rotate the patient under the operating microscope after laser capsulotomy and continue with the more "conventional" part of the procedure. Two side port incisions are created manually with a paracentesis knife; the anterior chamber is stabilized with an ophthalmic viscosurgical device (OVD), for instance, Healon 1.0%. In most cases we use the dimple-down technique described earlier. In this technique, a slight centripetal pressure on the capsule leads to the separation of the few potential remaining tags, and the anterior capsulotomy becomes completely free. The lens and cortex are removed with a bimanual irrigation/aspiration (I/A) device (Geuder AG). Next it is back under the laser: redocking is followed by the posterior capsulotomy. The final step takes place under the microscope again: In children younger than 3 years, we perform an anterior 23-gauge vitrectomy through the paracentesis and then close the incisions with 11-0 nylon sutures.

With growing experience we found out that particularly in very young children the capsulotomy diameter tends to turn out larger than planned. To correct for that aberration, we developed what is now known as the Bochum formula. According to this age-depending correction formula, the capsulotomy diameter in mm is to be programmed into the laser system's software:

$$\text{programmed diameter} = \frac{\text{aimed diameter}}{\left(1.34 + \left(-0.009 * \text{age}\right)\right)}$$

The Bochum formula for pediatric laser capsulotomies helps to minimize the age-depending deviation from the targeted diameter [15]. The anterior and posterior laser capsulotomy in children is, according to our experience, safe to perform. Implant IOLs was primarily in children 1 year and older, while secondary implantation was generally planned before the age of 6 years.

The operation is the first step to visual recovery for a child with cataract, to be followed by long-term care provided by the ophthalmologist. The parents (or caretakers) must be educated about the need for continuous follow-up so that complications like inflammation, glaucoma, and PCO can be detected and treated as soon as they arise, refractive errors can be corrected and amblyopia therapy pursued. In the immediate postoperative stage, the parents have to take care to administer pharmacological therapy as recommended by the surgeon or the ophthalmologist in charge of the follow-up. Normally, three different kinds of drugs are instilled as eye drops: antibiotics, anti-inflammatory agents, and maybe mydriatics/cycloplegics.

Antibiotics like fluoroquinolones are generally given for about a week after surgery, in regimens like every 6 h. This group of antibiotics is generally well tolerated; Ciprofloxacin is reported to have minimal adverse systemic side effects and is well tolerated by the corneal endothelium. Fourth-generation fluoroquinolones such as gatifloxacin and moxifloxacin have been successfully employed in children undergoing cataract surgery, both pre- and postoperatively.

Since the inflammatory response to cataract surgery might be quite intense in children, the frequent administration of topical and sometimes even systemic steroids is crucial to reduce the risk of complications like fibrinous membrane formation, synechia, the formation of inflammatory deposits on the IOL, and cystoid macular edema. Topical administration can mean the application of eye drops like 1% prednisolone acetate every 1–6 h or – in extreme cases – the subconjunctival injection of 2–4 mg dexamethasone. Depending on the patient's clinical presentation, the topical application of steroids – certainly the most common form of postoperative anti-inflammatory therapy – will be continued for up to 12 weeks. In cases where steroid-related complications like delayed wound healing or IOP rise are an issue, NSAID like diclofenac or ketorolac eye drops can be used. The rationale behind the postoperative administration of mydriatics and cycloplegics is pain reduction by dilating the pupil, preventing inflammation, stabilizing the blood-aqueous barrier, and diminishing the risk of synechia, pupillary block, and ciliary spasm.

Since a child's refractive status frequently changes during the first years of life, examinations are recommended every 2–3 months. Bifocal glasses for these children without accommodation are usually not tolerated before age 5 or 6. Particularly in younger children with an IOL, a considerable myopic shift can be expected [16].

Treating a child with cataract should give the cataract surgeon cause for a small pause in his or her daily routine, a short break in a sometimes overburdening schedule, and an incentive for some reflections: the child just operated upon will carry the marks of our intervention far into the future. The boy or girl of today will during a lifetime of many decades be treated not just by the next generation of ophthalmologists but also by the generation after the next one. They will have to deal with our success in BIL cataract surgery – and also with our failures.

14.6 Core Message

The femtosecond laser has been used successfully in thousands of cataract operations worldwide – in routine procedures but also in a wide variety of complicated cases like patients with corneal disease (Fuchs dystrophy, cornea guttata), intumescent cataract, small pupil, traumatic cataract, pediatric cataract, and Marfan syndrome. Its value for BIL cataract surgery is evident: the capsulotomies performed by the laser are of perfect circularity, optimal centration, and a diameter that fits the requirement of any IOL type chosen by the patient and the surgeon. Posterior capsulotomy, a step so crucial in BIL technique, is as reliably performed with the laser as it is so often manually demanding if not, in some cases, outright impossible. There is hardly any PCO and the alignment of the IOL promises to last for a lifetime – which in the case of children with cataract means many decades. The safety standard of the technique is high, complications are rare. Femtosecond laser BIL cataract surgery is a procedure which promises optimal results for many patients.

References

1. Manning S, Barry P, Henry Y, et al. Femtosecond laser-assisted cataract surgery versus standard phacoemulsification cataract surgery: study from the European registry of quality outcomes for cataract and refractive surgery. J Cataract Refract Surg. 2016;42:1779–90.
2. Day AC, Gore DM, Bunce C et al. Laser-assisted cataract surgery versus standard ultrasound phacoemulsification cataract surgery. Cochrane Database Of Systematic Reviews 2016, Issue 7. Art. No.: CD010735. 2016.
3. Conrad-Hengerer I, Al Juburi M, Schultz T, et al. Corneal endothelial cell loss and corneal thickness in conventional compared with femtosecond laser-assisted cataract surgery: three-month follow-up. J Cataract Refract Surg. 2013;39:1307–13.

4. Popovic M, Campos-Möller X, Schlenker MB, et al. Efficacy and safety of femtosecond laser-assisted cataract surgery compared with manual cataract surgery: a meta-analysis of 14567 eyes. Ophthalmology. 2016;123:2113–26.
5. Mastropasqua L, Toto L, Mastropasqua A, et al. Femtosecond laser versus manual clear corneal incision in cataract surgery. J Refract Surg. 2014;30:27–33.
6. Grewal DS, Schultz T, Basti S, Dick HB. Femtosecond laser-assisted cataract surgery - current status and future directions. Surv Ophthalmol. 2016;61:103–31.
7. Dick HB, Conrad-Hengerer I, Schultz T. Intraindividual capsular bag shrinkage comparing standard and laser-assisted cataract surgery. J Refract Surg. 2014;30:228–33.
8. Werner L, Tassignon M-J, Gobin L, et al. Bag-in-the-lens: first pathological analysis of a human eye obtained postmortem. J Cataract Refract Surg. 2008;34:2163–5.
9. Dick HB, Gerste RD, Schultz T, et al. Capsulotomy or capsulorhexis in femtosecond laser-assisted cataract surgery? J Cataract Refract Surg. 2013;39:1442.
10. Tassignon MJ, Gobin L, Mathysen D, et al. Clinical outcomes of cataract surgery after bag-in-the-lens intraocular lens implantation following ISO standard. J Cataract Refract Surg. 2011;37:2120–9.
11. Dick HB, Canto AP, Culbertson WW, et al. Femtosecond laser-assisted technique for performing bag-in-the-lens intraocular lens implantation. J Cataract Refract Surg. 2013;39:1286–90.
12. Schultz T, Joachim SC, Kuehn M, Dick HB. Changes in prostaglandin levels in patients undergoing femtosecond laser-assisted cataract surgery. J Refract Surg. 2013;29:742–7.
13. Dick HB, Gerste RD. Plea for femtosecond laser pretreatment and cataract surgery in the same room. J Cataract Refract Surg. 2014;40:499–500.
14. Dick HB, Gerste RD, Schultz T. Catalys precision laser systems. In: Guladi F, editor. Femtolaser cataract surgery. New Delhi: Jaypee; 2014. p. 167–74.
15. Dick HB, Schelenz D, Schultz T. Femtosecond laser-assisted pediatric cataract surgery: Bochum formula. J Cataract Refract Surg. 2015;41:821–6.
16. Dick HB, Schultz T. Femtosecond laser-assisted cataract surgery in infants. J Cataract Refract Surg. 2013;39:665–8.

Part III

Complex Cases

The Small Pupil

15

Luc Van Os

15.1 Introduction

Cataract surgery in eyes with small pupils can be very challenging to the surgeon. The visualization of the lens can be greatly diminished which will make every step of the surgery more difficult, from the anterior capsulorhexis to the positioning of the lens. As a consequence, surgery through a small pupil increases the risk of complications like iris damage, capsular tears with vitreous loss, etc. In the bag-in-the-lens technique, a small pupil can be a particular nuisance because of the importance of the correct sizing of both the anterior and posterior capsulorhexis. The positioning of the implant in the rhexis ring formed by the anterior and posterior rhexis is also more difficult when the pupillary aperture is small. In this chapter, we will elaborate on techniques used to facilitate safe surgery and the positioning of a bag-in-the-lens implant in eyes with small, poorly dilating pupils.

15.2 Surgical Technique

15.2.1 Preoperative Measures

Risk Identification

Small pupils are a common occurrence during cataract surgery; one study reported an incidence of 11% in uncomplicated cataract surgery [1]. Several subgroups of patients are known to be at risk for poor pupillary dilation (Table 15.1). It is

Electronic Supplementary Material The online version of this chapter (https://doi.org/10.1007/978-3-030-03086-5_15) contains supplementary material, which is available to authorized users.

L. Van Os (✉)
Department of Ophthalmology, Antwerp University, University Hospital, Edegem, Belgium
e-mail: luc.vanos@uza.be

M.-J. Tassignon et al. (eds.), *Innovative Implantation Technique*,
https://doi.org/10.1007/978-3-030-03086-5_15

important to be aware of these risk factors when assessing the patient during the preoperative visit. In pseudoexfoliation syndrome, the accumulation of fibrillar material in the iris results in a dysfunction of both the iris dilator and sphincter muscles [2]. Diabetes mellitus is another well-known risk factor for poor reaction to mydriatics [3]. This might be related to damages to the autonomous nervous system in patients with long-standing diabetes.

Anterior uveitis can result in the formation of posterior synechiae (Fig. 15.1), which will impede the pupil's dilation. Another mechanism causing miosis in patients with a history of uveitis is the formation of membranes on the pupillary border that also counteract the dilation of the pupil.

Intraoperative floppy iris syndrome (IFIS) is a triad of increased iris billowing, a tendency for iris prolapse through the incision and progressive miosis in the course of surgery. It is mainly related to the use of alpha-1A blockers such as tamsulosin, but it can also be caused by other drugs such as finasteride or certain antipsychotics. IFIS can still occur even if the patient discontinued the medication years before their surgery [4]. The chronic use of miotics can also result in decreased action of mydriatics. Finally, elderly patients frequently have smaller pupils than younger patients, which might be caused by a decrease in sympathetic activity.

Table 15.1 Risk factors for poorly dilating pupils

Pseudoexfoliation syndrome (PEX)
Diabetes mellitus
Intraoperative floppy iris syndrome (IFIS)
Uveitis
Chronic use of miotics
Elderly patients

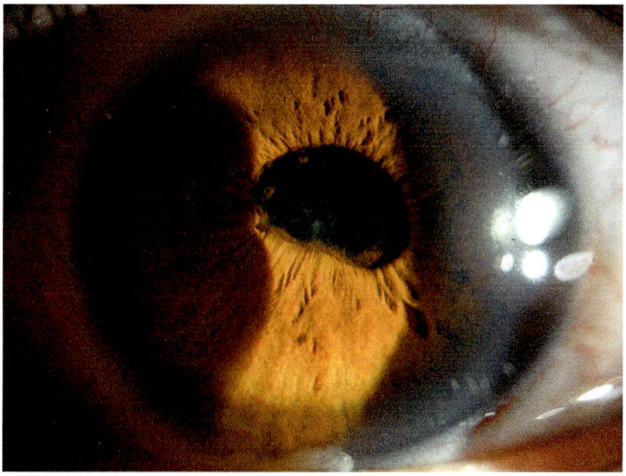

Fig. 15.1 Anterior segment photo illustrating posterior synechiae

Topical Mydriatics

A number of different mydriatics are currently available and can be divided into two groups according to their course of action. The first are the adrenergic stimulants that act through the stimulation of the iris dilator muscle, the most commonly used of which is phenylephrine. The second group consists of the parasympaticolytics (tropicamide, cyclopentolate, atropine) that result in inhibition of the iris sphincter muscle. When combined, their different modes of action will be complementary and result in maximum pupillary dilation.

The formulations can be administered in the form of eye drops (e.g. tropicamide 5 mg/ml, phenylephrine 10%) or in the form of an ocular insert containing both tropicamide and phenylephrine that can be positioned in the inferior fornix 1 h prior to surgery (Mydriasert, Laboratoires Théa, France).

Topical NSAIDs

Nonsteroidal anti-inflammatory drugs (NSAIDs) block cyclooxygenases 1 and 2 (COX 1, COX2), resulting in a decreased transformation of arachidonic acid to prostaglandins. Prostaglandins cause smooth muscle contraction in the iris and are thus involved in miosis [5]. As a consequence, the preoperative use of topical NSAID can help in sustaining mydriasis throughout the surgery [6]. In our centre, we use topical diclofenac 1 mg/ml (Dicloabak®, Laboratoires Théa, France), one drop, every 15 min, for 1 h prior to surgery.

15.2.2 Intraoperative Measures

Intracameral Mydriatics

To obtain additional mydriasis at the start of surgery, intracameral administration of mydriatics can be used. Several different preparations have been used and proven to be safe, e.g. adrenaline, phenylephrine, ketorolac, etc. In our centre we now use a commercially available solution of tropicamide, phenylephrine and lidocaine (Mydrane®, Laboratoires Théa, France) at the start of the surgery to assist in mydriasis and pain control. Previously we used a mixture of adrenaline 1/1000 with lidocaine. Intracameral injection will provide a more stable iris and a more sustained dilation than topical mydriatics [7].

Viscoelastics

Using a cohesive ophthalmic viscosurgical device (OVD) will also aid in dilating the pupil further. However, when there is very little reaction to the mydriatics already administered, it is not likely to be sufficient to allow to proceed with the bag-in-the-lens procedure comfortably. In this case, it would be advisable to use a pupil expanding device.

Lysis of Synechiae and Membranes

The pupil will not dilate in case of the presence of posterior synechiae because of the adhesion of the iris tissue to the anterior lens capsule. When these are disengaged, it can result in immediate and sufficient mydriasis without the need for the further use of surgical devices in some cases.

The separation of posterior synechiae is obtained through viscodissection (Fig. 15.2, Video 15.1) with an OVD and through the use of a blunt spatula if necessary.

In addition to posterior synechiae, membranes on the pupillary margin can impede the pupil to fully dilate. They are mostly the result of anterior chamber inflammation and can be seen in patients with a history of uveitis. These can be removed by peeling them off the pupillary edge with a fine-toothed forceps, like the Ikeda microforceps (Fr2268 EyeTech) which we also use to perform the capsulorhexis.

Pupil Expansion Ring

We prefer to use a pupil expansion ring in case dilation after topical and intracameral administration of mydriatics is insufficient, and any present synechiae or membranes are removed. In our centre, we use the Malyugin ring (MicroSurgical Technology (MST), USA) with a diameter of 7 mm, given that smaller diameters will not accommodate the BIL. Other pupil expansion rings are available; each type of these devices has its own advantages and disadvantages. In case of bag-in-the-lens surgery, it is, however, important that the size of the ring is big enough, due to the design of the IOL. This is why we use the 7 mm Malyugin ring rather than the 6.25 mm, to provide sufficient space to insert the implant through the newly created pupillary opening.

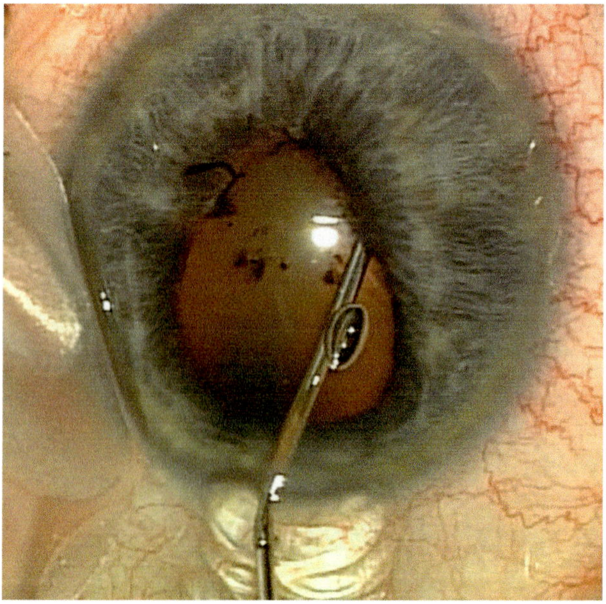

Fig. 15.2 Viscodissection of posterior synechiae

The Malyugin ring is very valuable in cataract surgery in eyes at risk of intra-operative floppy iris syndrome (IFIS). It will prevent the iris from progressively becoming miotic through the course of the surgery and will provide a more stable iris. Iris prolapse can still occur, but it will be less frequent and easier to reposition [8].

The Malyugin ring comes preloaded with an injector which makes its positioning quite straightforward (Video 15.2). The plunger on the device must first be slid back to load the ring. Then the tip of the injector device is inserted through the main incision of at least 2.2 mm. The first scroll of the ring will appear when the plunger is slid forward. This should be led towards the opposite edge of the pupil where the scroll will catch the iris between both coils of the scroll. The ring is then further injected into the anterior chamber. The three remaining scrolls can be positioned by using a blunt hooked instrument, such as a Lester manipulator.

After positioning the ring, the pupillary aperture will be large enough to continue the surgery following the usual protocol. As mentioned previously, great care should be taken when positioning the bag in the lens. The haptics can catch the iris or the ring itself and make implantation more difficult because of the design of the lens. Therefore, after injecting the lens into the eye, start by carefully positioning the IOL behind the iris but in front of the capsular bag (Fig. 15.3). This way the iris will not be able to hinder further positioning when sliding the capsule edges into the

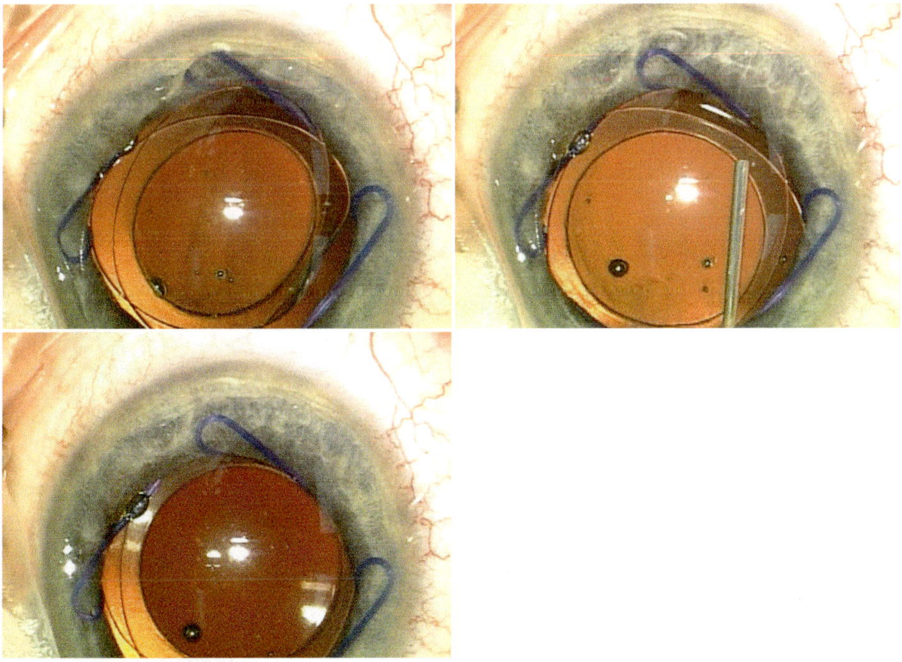

Fig. 15.3 Gently manipulating the BIL through the Malyugin ring stepwise

peripheral groove of the IOL. After the IOL has been properly placed, the Malyugin ring can be removed from the eye by disengaging the scrolls.

Iris Retraction Hooks
Iris retraction hooks are a helpful adjunct to the surgery if a pupil expansion ring is not available or if the pupil is too small to enable the use of one. Care should be taken in the positioning of each of the hooks so that insertion and positioning of the IOL is not hindered later on in the surgery.

15.3 Complications

When preparing solutions for intracameral injection, care should be taken to avoid contamination that could result in toxic anterior segment syndrome (TASS) or endophthalmitis.

Using pupil expansion devices can result in iris damage or tissue loss and transillumination and sometimes permanent mydriasis. However, these complications are very rare with the currently available pupil expansion devices.

15.4 Core Messages

- Identify patients at risk for poor dilation.
- Try to ensure proper mydriasis before surgery.
- If in doubt or unstable iris, do not hesitate to use a pupil expansion ring (e.g. Malyugin ring).
- Take care positioning the implant – start close to the capsule surface to avoid trapping the iris.

15.5 Instruments Used

The instruments listed are our preference, but similar ones can be used based on the surgeon's own preference.

Item	Description	Manufacturer
OVD	Healon GV	Abbott Medical Optics, USA
Microforceps	Ikeda angled 30° capsulorhexis 23.0 g forceps	EyeTech Fr2268
Malyugin ring 7,0 mm	Pupil expansion ring	MicroSurgical Technology, USA

References

1. Hashemi H, Mohammadpour M, Jabbarvand M, Nezamdoost Z, Ghadimi H. Incidence of and risk factors for vitreous loss in resident-performed phacoemulsification surgery. J Cataract Refract Surg. 2013;39:1377–82.
2. Repo LP, Naukkarinen A, Paljärvi L, Teräsvirta ME. Pseudoexfoliation syndrome with poorly dilating pupil: a light and electron microscopic study of the sphincter area. Graefes Arch Clin Exp Ophthalmol. 1996;234:171–6.
3. Lei HL, Yang KJ, Sun CC, Chen CH, Huang BY, Ng SC, Yeung L. Obtained mydriasis in long-term type 2 diabetic patients. J Ocul Pharmacol Ther. 2011;27:599–602.
4. Abdel-Aziz S, Mamalis N. Intraoperative floppy iris syndrome. Curr Opin Ophthalmol. 2009;20:37–40.
5. Hoffman RS, Braga-Mele R, Donaldson K, Emerick G, Henderson B, Kahook M, Mamalis N, Miller KM, Realini T, Shorstein NH, Stiverson RK, Wirostko B. Cataract surgery and nonsteroidal antiinflammatory drugs. J Cataract Refract Surg. 2016;42:1368–79.
6. Mishima S, Tanishima T, Masuda K. Pathophysiology and pharmacology of intraocular surgery. Aust N Z J Ophthalmol. 1985;13:147–58.
7. Lundqvist O, Koskela T, Behndig A. A paired comparison of intracameral mydriatics in refractive lens exchange surgery. Acta Ophthalmol. 2014;92:482–5.
8. Chang DF. Use of Malyugin pupil expansion device for intraoperative floppy-iris syndrome: results in 30 consecutive cases. J Cataract Refract Surg. 2008;34:835–41.

BIL in Patients with Uveitis

16

Christian Billotte

16.1 Introduction

Cataracts are a very frequent complication associated with chronic uveitis and long-term corticosteroid therapy. Different aetiologies are responsible, but patients with uveitis and cataract often have common characteristics. The cataract occurs at a younger age than in the typical cataract, and they often have impaired pupillary dilation with the added complexity of posterior synechiae (PS). These cataracts can also opacify quickly and result in significant visual impairment. Different manifestations of lens opacification have been observed, but there is a high rate of posterior capsular opacification and white cataract. Ocular hypertension is also frequent in uveitis, and this can be due to the chronic inflammation as such or secondary to the anti-inflammatory medication.

Cystoid macular oedema can also be present in a high percentage of patients and should be looked for during the preoperative assessment, either by OCT imaging or clinical evaluation. When planning the cataract surgery itself, a three-month period of uveitis quiescence is advised. We also recommend an increase in the anti-inflammatory treatment at least 1 week prior to surgery. The current international standard of care is phacoemulsification surgery followed by the implantation of a lens in the bag acrylic IOL. While successful, this approach is associated with secondary complications [1–5] due to postoperative inflammation and the important participation of the epithelial cells of the lens capsule in particular in this

Electronic Supplementary Material The online version of this chapter (https://doi.org/10.1007/978-3-030-03086-5_16) contains supplementary material, which is available to authorized users.

C. Billotte (✉)
CHU of Caen, Caen, France
e-mail: billotte@fondation-misericorde.fr

M.-J. Tassignon et al. (eds.), *Innovative Implantation Technique*,
https://doi.org/10.1007/978-3-030-03086-5_16

inflammatory environment. These secondary complications include capsular bag contraction, IOL displacement, rapid secondary opacification of the visual axis, cystoid macular oedema [4–7] and hypertony [8]. These complications may require further medication, secondary intervention or Nd:YAG capsulotomy.

16.2 Impaired Pupillary Dilation

Impaired pupillary dilation is very common in uveitis, but it is never an intractable situation. The first thing to do is to inject some mydriatic agent in the anterior chamber, in the vicinity of the irido-capsular synechiae. Under ocular viscoelatic device (OVD) coverage, release the synechiae mechanically with a Lester hook or similar tool (Figs. 16.1 and 16.2). An additional corneal paracentesis may help in this. The reinjection of cohesive OVD will, most of the time, allow at least 5 mm pupil diameter, a necessity for the BIL procedure (Fig. 16.3), to be inserted and to centre the 5 mm calliper to size the anterior capsulorhexis (Fig. 16.4).

While we try to avoid touching the iris, in some cases, mechanical pupil maintainers, such as a Malyugin ring (Figs. 16.5, 16.6 and 16.7) or equivalent cannot be avoided. We tend to use iris retractors (Figs. 16.8, 16.9 and 16.10) though this requires four paracenteses. The advantage of the pupillary ring over iris hooks is better stabilization as iris hooks can sometimes herniate through the uveitic iris due to its weakness. Malyugin rings are available in a variety of sizes but it is important to note that if you choose a 6 mm diameter ring, it is very difficult to fit the BIL through the ring, given that its total width is 7.5 mm. In these cases, it is easier to

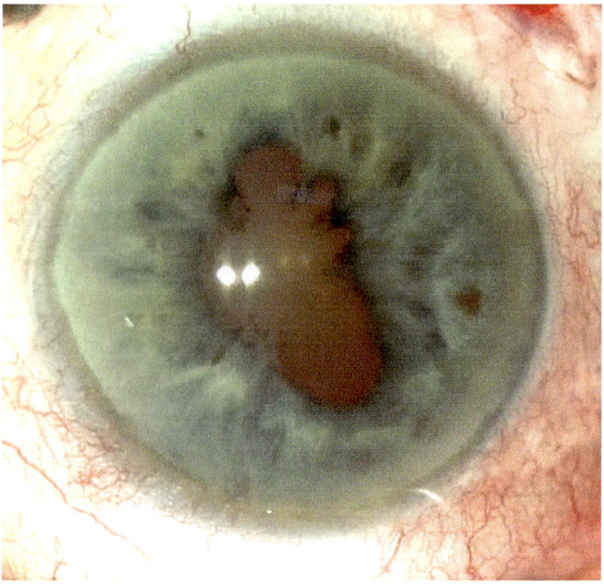

Fig. 16.1 Uveitic eye with posterior synechiae

just remove the ring prior to lens injection. Reinjection of OVD is usually enough to maintain the pupil diameter during implantation. The BIL can be implanted through a 7 mm Malyugin ring. In that case it is not necessary to remove the ring until after BIL implantation. The surgeon must decide about the best ring size based on the patient's eye condition. Other solutions such as iris stretching, iridotomies and sphincterotomies are more traumatic to the iris tissues, and I do not tend to use them. Iris retractors can be very useful under the right circumstances.

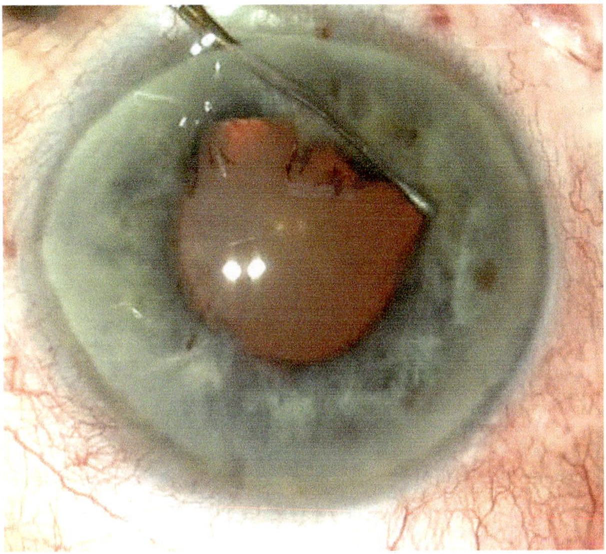

Fig. 16.2 Manual dissection of posterior synechiae with a Lester hook

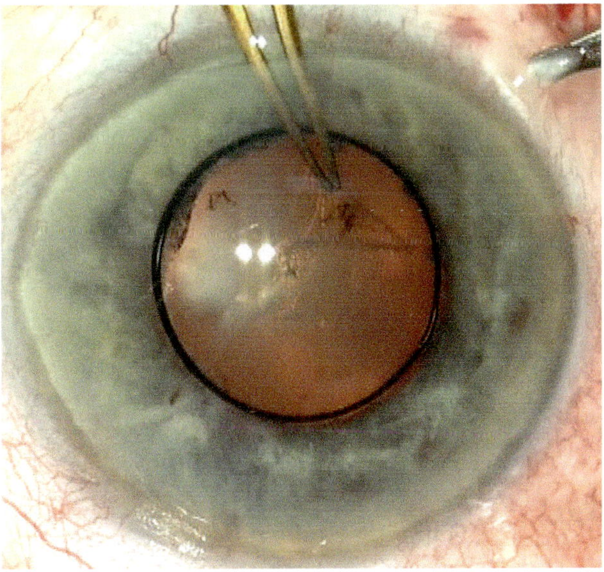

Fig. 16.3 Performing a posterior rhexis through a 5 mm pupil

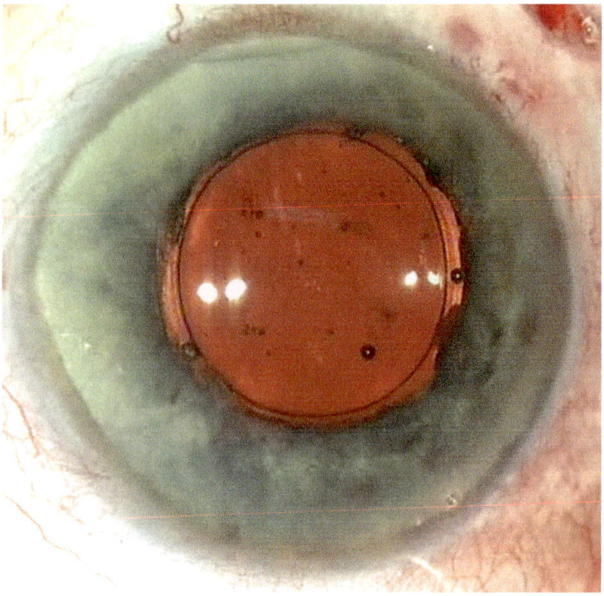

Fig. 16.4 The BIL in place

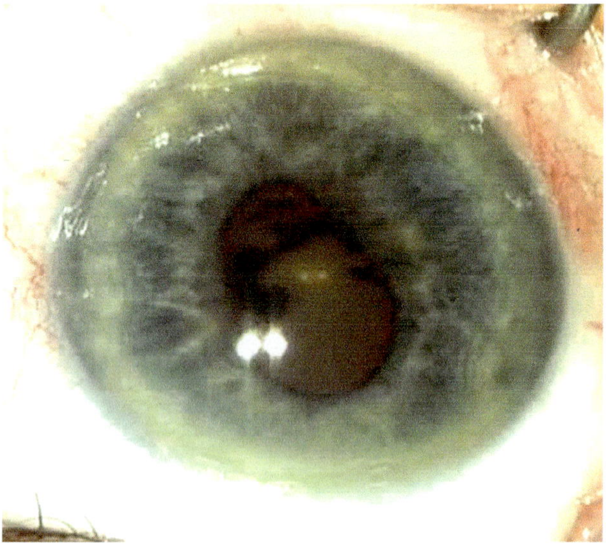

Fig. 16.5 Uveitic eye with posterior synechiae

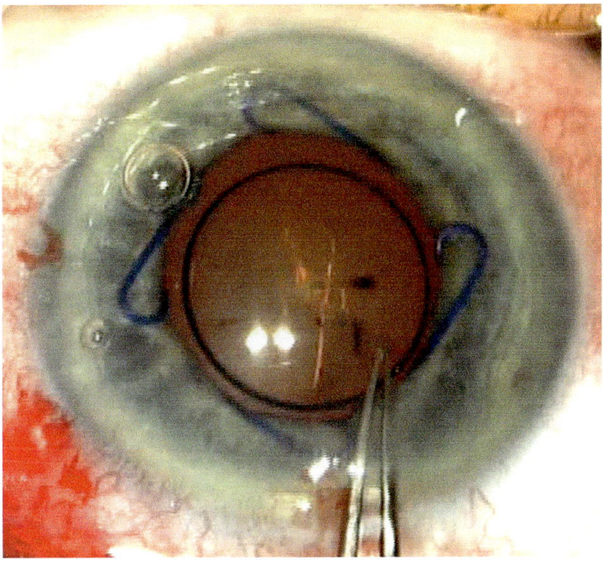

Fig. 16.6 Performing an anterior rhexis through a Malyugin ring

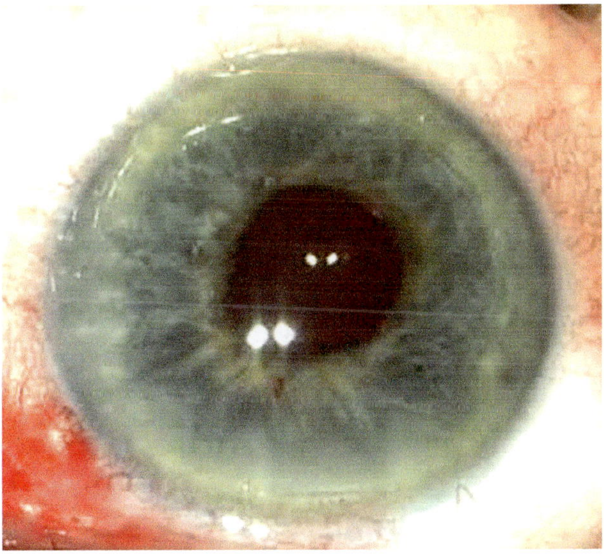

Fig. 16.7 The BIL in a uveitis case

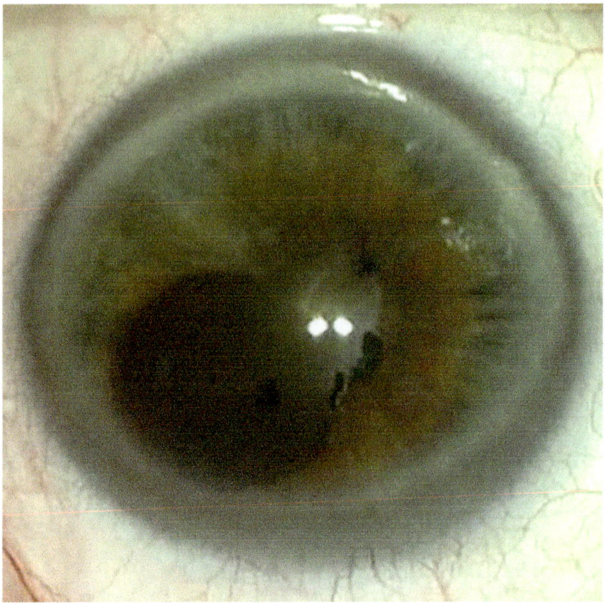

Fig. 16.8 Uveitic eye preoperatively

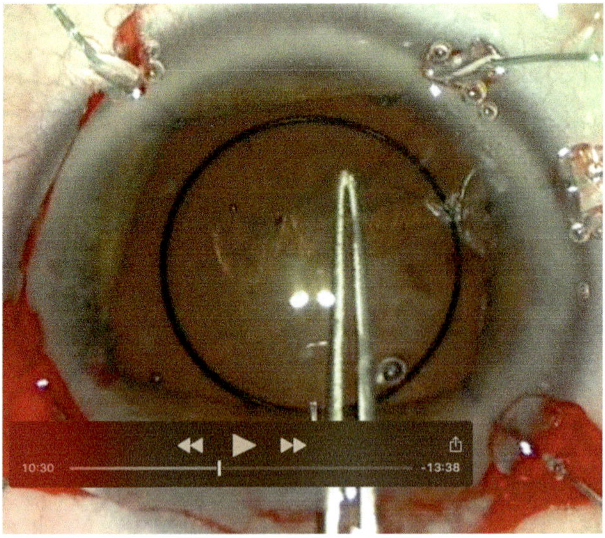

Fig. 16.9 Iris hooks in the uveitic eye

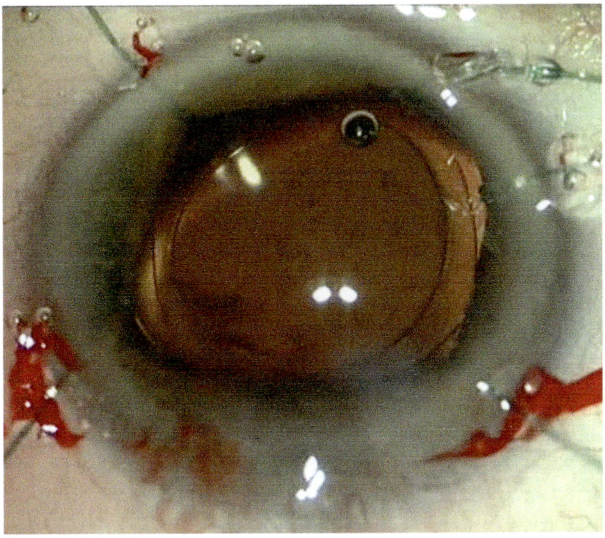

Fig. 16.10 The BIL in place under four iris hooks

16.3 Anterior Capsulorhexis

The circular capsulotomy can be performed with great care, as described in a previous chapter, once the pupil diameter has reached a minimum of 5 mm. Patients with uveitis can often present with a white or intumescent cataract. In these cases, we recommend the use of trypan blue to stain the capsule as an accurate capsulorhexis is key in the BIL technique. The role of the femtosecond laser in these cases has not yet been fully evaluated, but we are not convinced that it adds value. It can also present other risks, particularly in cases with small pupils. If you do choose to perform femtolaser in these cases, it should also be adapted because the anterior capsule tends to be thicker and great care is needed to avoid the iris.

16.4 Phakoemulsification

The visibility of the posterior capsule can be reduced so hydrodissection should also be undertaken with care. The posterior capsule can also be very fragile and may break more easily. The phacoemulsification itself is not the most demanding stage of the procedure, given that these cataracts occur in younger patients and the lens can be softer. It can also be helpful to perform the cortex material removal using a bimanual approach. All cortical material and strands should be removed to improve capsule visibility for the posterior capsulorhexis to be performed as next step.

The primary posterior continuous curvilinear capsulorhexis is performed as in all cases of BIL cataract surgery. Cohesive OVD helps greatly to maintain a pupil diameter that is sufficient to make the posterior CCC of the same size as the anterior. If the posterior rhexis is too small, then it can be enlarged like an anterior rhexis.

This is done by making a small snip in the edge of the rhexis with retinal scissors. The capsulorhexis can then be enlarged without compromising the strength of the capsule. If the PPCCC is larger than the anterior rhexis, the lens will be fine, as anterior rhexis can support the BIL alone. If the ACCC is too large though, then the posterior CCC should be performed with great accuracy in order to promote BIL stability.

The lens is injected into the anterior chamber over the level of the iris. If the pupil is too small, you may need to use a two-handed technique to insert the lens and retract the iris at the same time (Video 16.1). It is essential that the groove of the BIL is visible when inserting the lens to confirm that it has been placed correctly. The pupil tends to be smaller in these cases, so the pupil constriction required in other BIL cases is usually not needed once the remaining OVD has been removed.

We complete these cases with a sub-tenon injection of long-acting triamcinolone. The postoperative care consists of NSAID drops and a combination of corticosteroids drops with antibiotics. Drops are given four to six times a day, depending on the clinical case. We do not recommend mydriatic drops postoperatively as this can result in iris incarceration in the BIL. Systemic medication is adapted based on the underlying uveitis and postoperative clinical findings.

16.5 Managing Complications

If the anterior rhexis is lost, then a traditional lens-in-the-bag technique can be used. If they are available, bean-shaped ring segments can recreate the rhexis opening and allow the BIL to be used in these cases. If the posterior capsule is torn during the phacoemulsification with vitreous loss, the BIL can still be used. The surgeon can choose to insert a sulcus lens, but for those more familiar with the BIL implantation, the lens can be inserted and suspended only by the anterior capsulorhexis.

In all cases with uveitis, it is important to carefully evaluate the zonular integrity and stability of the natural crystalline lens prior to surgery and/or during surgery. If zonular integrity is weak, the BIL is more prone to anterior displacement and iris capture. If this is likely to happen, the best course of action is to create a peripheral iridotomy. It is therefore also mandatory to ensure wound closure by means of hydration or with sutures.

16.6 Advantages of BIL in Uveitis

Measuring postoperative inflammation is often difficult in uveitis. There are so many different aetiologies clustered under the collective term uveitis, which a one-size-fits-all approach is not possible. A multicentre clinical approach is needed in order to compare lens-in-the-bag and bag-in-the-lens implantation. Until a broader evidence base has been established, we can only speak from our years of clinical experience with the BIL. It is our clinical experience that postoperative inflammation is very low. This is a general observation, not only in uveitis but also in eyes at risk of postoperative inflammation, e.g. diabetes, capsular exfoliation, children and combined posterior segment surgery.

The sealed closure of the equator of the bag prevents the reaction of the lens epithelial cells with the biomaterial of the IOL. It also prevents the release of cells and inflammatory mediators into the aqueous humour factors. The remaining peripheral part of the capsular bag will guarantee perfect centration and stable refraction, provided that both anterior and posterior CCC have been well-performed and the zonules are solid. We had one case of pupil block that did not generate a raised intraocular pressure despite not having an iridotomy. We believe that this was due to iris atrophy.

The eradication of secondary cataract is easier to measure. In our series of 51 uveitic eyes, the rate of secondary cataract was 0%, and no anterior capsular phimosis was observed. The absence of secondary YAG capsulotomies also prevents all of the complications after posterior YAG-laser capsulotomy and no patient presented a dislocation of the BIL IOL.

Other situations, such as combined phako-vitrectomy, usually carry a high risk of secondary inflammation, leading to posterior iris synechiae, early anterior and posterior capsular opacification and contraction. In a study by Auchere-Lavayssière [9] comparing 45 patients of phako-vitrectomy with BIL (group 1) and 55 with LIB (group 2), posterior iris synechiae and capsular modifications were checked after at least 3 months of observation. The occurrence of posterior synechiae was significantly reduced ($p = 0{,}003$) in group 1 BIL (2%), versus (40%) in group 2 LIB. In 45 patients of phako-vitrectomy with BIL (group 1) and 55 with LIB (group 2), posterior iris synechiae and capsular modifications were checked after at least 3 months of observation.

PCO needing YAG capsulotomy occurred in 0% in group BIL versus 36% in group LIB ($p < 0{,}0001$). No anterior capsular phimosis occurred in group BIL, compared to 11% in group LIB. These results show a dramatic decrease in the side effects related to postoperative inflammation with the BIL.

16.7 Summary

In our experience of almost 10 years, the IOL implantation with the bag-in-the-lens gives much better results in every situation of inflammation, than classical in the bag IOL implantation.

Acknowledgements C Auchère-Vayssière, G Bois, E Denion, E Grée

References

1. Llop SM, Papaliodis GN. Cataract surgery complications in uveitis patients: a review article. Semin Ophthalmol. 2018;33(1):64–9.
2. Elgohary MA, Mc Cluskey PJ, Towler HM, Okhravi N, Singh RP, Obokpo R, Lightman SS. Outcome of phacoemulsification in patients with uveitis. Br J Ophthalmol. 2007;91(7):916–21.
3. Mehta S, Linton MM, Kempen JH. Outcomes of cataract surgery in patients with uveitis: a systematic review and meta-analysis. Am J Ophthalmol. 2014 Oct;158(4):676–92.

4. Yoeruek E, Deuter C, Gieselmann S, Saygili O, Spitzer MS, Tatar O, Bartz-Schmidt KU, Szurman P. Long-term visual acuity and its predictors after cataract surgery in patients with uveitis. Eur J. 2010;20(4):694–701. https://www.ncbi.nlm.nih.gov/pubmed/20213617.
5. Allio GL, Chipont E, Benezra D, Fakhry MA, IOS study group of uveitis. Comparative performance of intraocular lenses in eyes with cataract and uveitis. J Cataract Refract Surg. 2002;28:2096–108.
6. Lobo AM, Papaliodis GN. Perioperative evaluation and management of cataract surgery in uveitis patients. Int Ophthalmol Clin. 2010;50(1):129–37.
7. Bélair ML, Kim SJ, Thorne JE, Dunn JP, Kedhar SR, Brown DM, Jabs DA. Incidence of cystoid macular edema after cataract surgery in patients with and without uveitis using optical coherence tomography. Ophthalmology. 2009;148(1):128–35.
8. Friedman DS, Holbrook JT, Ansari H, Alexander J, Burke A, Reed SB, Katz J, Thorne JE, Lightman SL, Kempen JH, MUST Research Group. Risk of elevated intraocular pressure and glaucoma in patients with uveitis: results of the multicenter uveitis steroid treatment trial. Ophthalmology. 2013;120(8):1571–9.
9. Auchère Lavayssière C, Lux AL, Degoumois A, Billotte C, Denion E. Bag-in-the-lens implantation avoids posterior synechiae of the iris after phacovitrectomy. J Cataract Refract Surg. 2018. Submitted.

Zonulolysis and Lens Luxation

17

Nils-Erik Boonstra

17.1 Introduction

Zonulolysis is defined as a weak or absent zonular support of the lens capsule. This can result in malposition of the lens, either subluxation or total luxation of the lens. Zonulolysis and lens luxation are known challenges in cataract and lens surgery. Different techniques have been used and recommended, but to date no consensus has been reached on the best surgical approach [1]. Much depends on the surgeon's preference and experience.

The causes of zonulolysis are many, but some of the most common causes are associated with injuries (Fig. 17.1). In children and young adults, ectopia lentis is more likely to be associated with heritable conditions like Marfan syndrome, homocysteinuria and Weill-Marchesani syndrome [2, 3]. Ectopia lentis is also seen in more isolated conditions like mutation in the *ADAMTSL4* gene [4]. In the elderly, pseudoexfoliation syndrome is probably the most common cause of subluxation.

In the last two decades, there has been a continuous development of surgical techniques, intraocular lenses and supporting devices, enabling the surgeon to preserve the capsular bag rather than performing conventional intracapsular cataract extraction (ICCE) or a pars plana lensectomy. Preserving the capsular bag allows for the support of a posterior chamber intraocular lens (IOL), minimizes the risk of vitreous loss and reduces complications such as retinal detachment. Thus, ICCE and pars plana lensectomy with scleral or iris fixated intraocular lens are now more frequently regarded as backup measures.

Electronic Supplementary Material The online version of this chapter (https://doi.org/10.1007/978-3-030-03086-5_17) contains supplementary material, which is available to authorized users.

N.-E. Boonstra (✉)
Department of Ophthalmology, Haukeland University Hospital, Bergen, Norway
e-mail: nils-erik.boonstra@helse-bergen.no

M.-J. Tassignon et al. (eds.), *Innovative Implantation Technique*,
https://doi.org/10.1007/978-3-030-03086-5_17

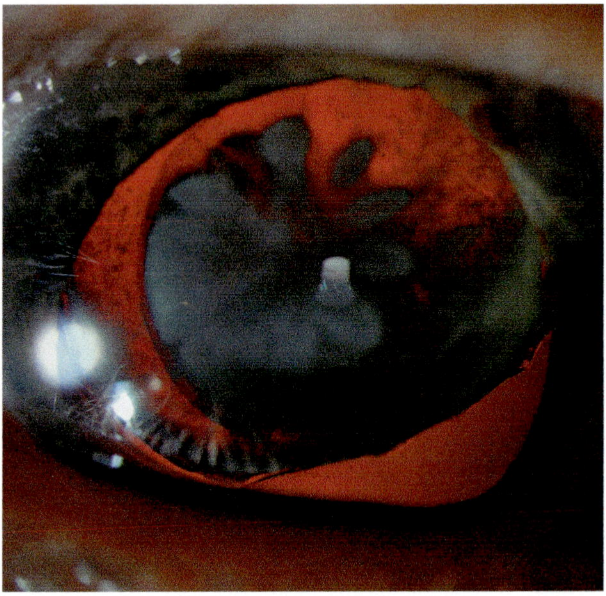

Fig. 17.1 Traumatic cataract and zonulolysis

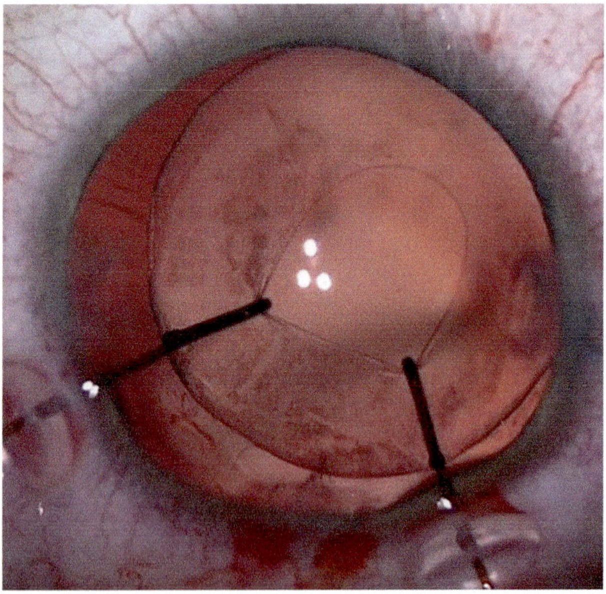

Fig. 17.2 Capsular hooks

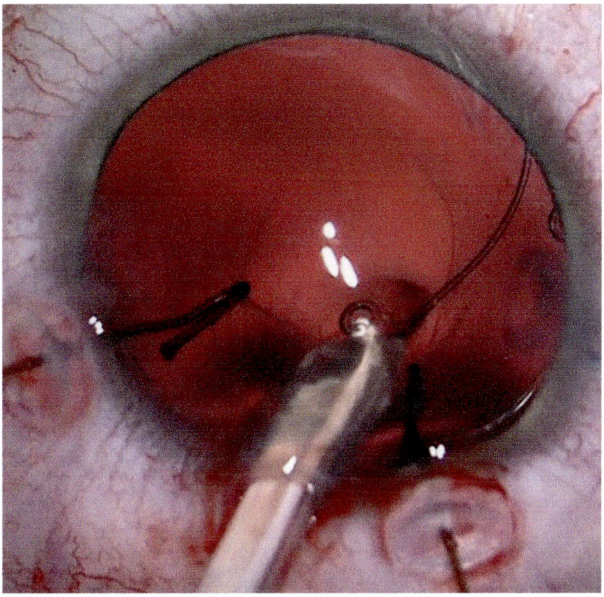

Fig. 17.3 Capsular hooks and capsular tension ring placement

Excellent and innovative techniques with different sutured supporting rings have been developed [5]. Cionni capsular tension ring and Ahmed capsular tension segment are used with traditional lens-in-the-bag (LIB) IOLs. Capsular hooks (Fig. 17.2) enable the surgeon to stabilize the capsular bag during lens and cortex removal, and capsular tension rings (CTR) (Fig. 17.3) expand the capsular bag and distribute the force to the remaining zonulas. However, over time the capsular bag may shrink, and sutures may break, both with possible re-subluxation of the lens needing additional surgery. In addition, posterior capsule opacities (PCO) probably occur more commonly due to an incomplete closure of the capsular bag. YAG capsulotomy may be difficult in these cases.

The bag-in-the-lens (BIL) IOL gives no PCO or capsular shrinking in front of the IOL [6]. Its design, with a central groove, allows it to be fixated to the sclera with *lasso suture(s)* (Fig. 17.4b) or by a non-suture technique using two specially developed *bean-shaped segments* (Fig. 17.4c) for both support and centration, neither interfering with the closed capsular bag. Together, this makes the BIL particularly suited for use in challenging cases with zonular weakness and lens luxation. This chapter describes both ways of fixation and centring the BIL in eyes with mild to severe lens luxation.

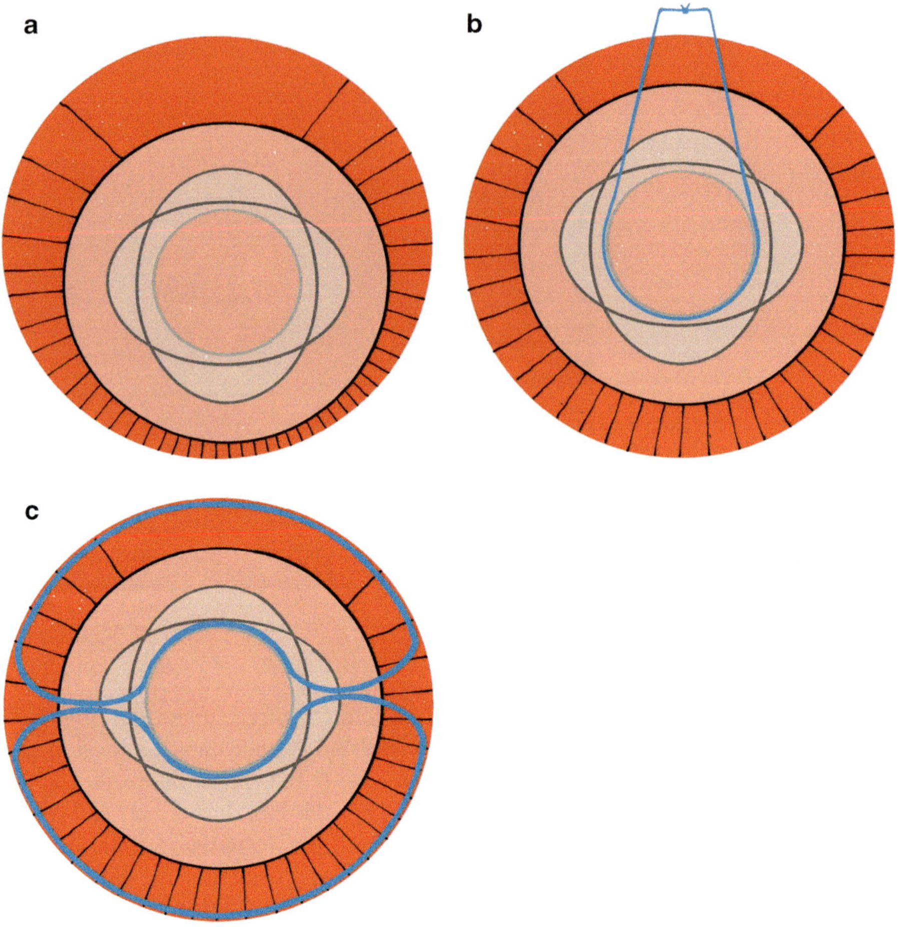

Fig. 17.4 Illustration of bag-in-the-lens after implantation in an eye with zonulolysis (**a**), after centration with "lasso suture" to the sclera (**b**) and after centration with two bean-shaped rings in the sulcus (**c**)

17.2 Methods

When dealing with challenging cases of zonulolysis, it is an advantage to master not only one but several of these techniques, given that different cases may profit from different approaches. The bag-in-the-lens is superior in preventing PCO and capsular shrinking. The two techniques described below show how one can centre and stabilize the "capsular bag – BIL" complex directly, without interfering with capsular integrity. Both techniques have also been used in children.

17.2.1 Lasso Suturing

In cases with mild subluxation of the lens, it may be sufficient to simply place a CTR to regain centration. However, if additional fixation seems necessary during surgery with lens-in-the-bag (LIB) and CTR, this cannot be done in the same operation because some degree of capsular fibrosis is needed before suturing through the capsular bag without the risk of creating a tear in the bag.

In LIB cases, where one wishes to fixate the IOL peroperatively, the choice stands between different fixation rings like the Cionni capsular tension ring or Ahmed capsular tension segment. This allows the capsular bag with IOL to be fixated to the sclera without suturing through the capsular bag and is useful to have in stock for special cases.

When using the bag-in-the-lens IOL, one has the possibility to "lasso" the IOL to the sclera by placing one or more sutures in the interhaptic groove of the lens. This allows for the direct suturing and centration of the IOL.

17.2.1.1 Surgical Technique

Surgery is performed under local anaesthesia, preferably retrobulbar. The pupil is dilated with cyclopentolate and phenylephrine preoperatively. A standard approach with two 1.2 mm side ports and a 2.2 mm main incision at the limbus is made. The anterior chamber is filled with Ophthalmic Viscosurgical Device (OVD) in softshell technique (Viscoat® and Provisc®). In cases with a small degree of lens subluxation, a capsulorhexis with the correct size is made using a caliper ring. Thorough hydrodissection allows for the rotation of the nucleus with less force on the remaining zonulas. Careful nucleus removal, preferably with chopping in dense cataract cases, is recommended. The cortex is removed with the irrigation-aspiration system. The capsular bag is filled with OVD (Provisc®), and a standard size CTR is placed. In more severe cases of zonulolysis, the CTR may have to be placed before or during lens removal (Fig. 17.5a). In some cases, capsular hooks may be needed. The OVD is removed from the capsular bag, and the anterior chamber is refilled with it. Alternatively, the CTR can be implanted without OVD in the capsular bag. A small tear centrally in the posterior capsule is made with a 30G needle, and Berger's space is filled up with OVD beyond the size of the capsulorhexis. A posterior capsulorhexis is made using a microforceps with the anterior rhexis as guide. If capsular hooks are used, these can be repositioned through both capsulorhexes if additional support is needed during lens implantation. The main incision is increased to 3.0 mm. The BIL 89A is injected into the anterior chamber and pushed into position close to the capsular bag. The posterior haptic is gently manipulated through both rhexes. If hooks are used, they should be removed during this procedure to facilitate the smooth edge of both rhexes to slip into the interhaptic groove. Depending on the design of the hooks, it may be possible to remove them after positioning the BIL.

Depending on the degree of the zonulolysis, either one or two lasso sutures should be placed. If needed, even more sutures can be placed, but extra stabilization can also be obtained by increasing the distance between the entry and the exit points of each suture. The scleral fixation should be at the place of maximum zonular weakness. An optional second lasso can be placed opposite to the first. The conjunctiva is recessed to facilitate scleral suturing at the pars plicata. The preferable suture is Prolene 9-0 with a straight needle, but other non-resorbable sutures may also be used. The OVD is injected into the sulcus at the place of suturing, and the needle is passed through the pars plicata into the sulcus 1.5 mm behind the limbus. The needle is met by a cannula through one of the limbal incisions and is externalized (Fig. 17.5b). It is then turned around and passed back through a 25G cannula placed through the pars plicata 2–5 mm from the first insertion point (Fig. 17.5c). The thread is guided into the interhaptic groove with the Y-manipulator or a similar tool (Fig. 17.5d). It may be necessary to do this bimanually with two instruments (Fig. 17.5e). The lasso should be tightened enough to allow good centration. After the knot is made, it should be rotated into the eye (Fig. 17.5f). Alternatively, the knot could be placed beneath a scleral flap or in a scleral pocket. An optional second "lasso suture" should be placed in the same manner on the opposite side. In cases of severe zonulolysis and risk of luxation of the capsular bag – IOL complex to the posterior pole during suturing – a temporary intended "iris capture" of the BIL can be useful. An iridectomy can be made in cases with a high risk of postoperative "iris capture" or pupillary block. The OVD is removed using the irrigation-aspiration system and the conjunctiva closed with Vicryl 8-0 resorbable sutures. Cefuroxime (Aprokam®) is installed in the anterior chamber at the end of surgery.

17.2.1.2 Complications of the "Lasso" Technique

- *Suture break*: One of the known complications of scleral suturing an IOL is breakage of the suture and dislocation of the IOL. This is probably also the case with "lasso suture" of the BIL. To prevent suture break, Prolene 9-0 or similar should be used with careful handling to avoid kinks during suturing.
- *Subluxation*: The IOL complex may subluxate, either due to suture break or progressive zonulolysis. Re-suturing should be considered if the degree of luxation affects vision or leads to other symptoms. This can be done with either new or additional lasso sutures or by suturing the CRT to the sclera in one or two locations.
- *Iris capture*: Iris capture may occur in cases with loose IOL complex or sutures placed too anteriorly. Treatment is either medical by dilating the pupil or surgical by repositioning the BIL. An iridotomy should be performed, preventing recapturing by deepening the anterior chamber.

17.2.2 Bean-Shaped Rings

Another way to centralize the BIL-IOL in cases of zonulolysis and lens luxation is by using the specially designed bean-shaped rings (Fig. 17.6). The insertion of the custom-designed bean-shaped ring was originally used intracapsularly in eyes with localized zonular defects, but they can also be placed in the sulcus for permanent non-sutured centration of the BIL.

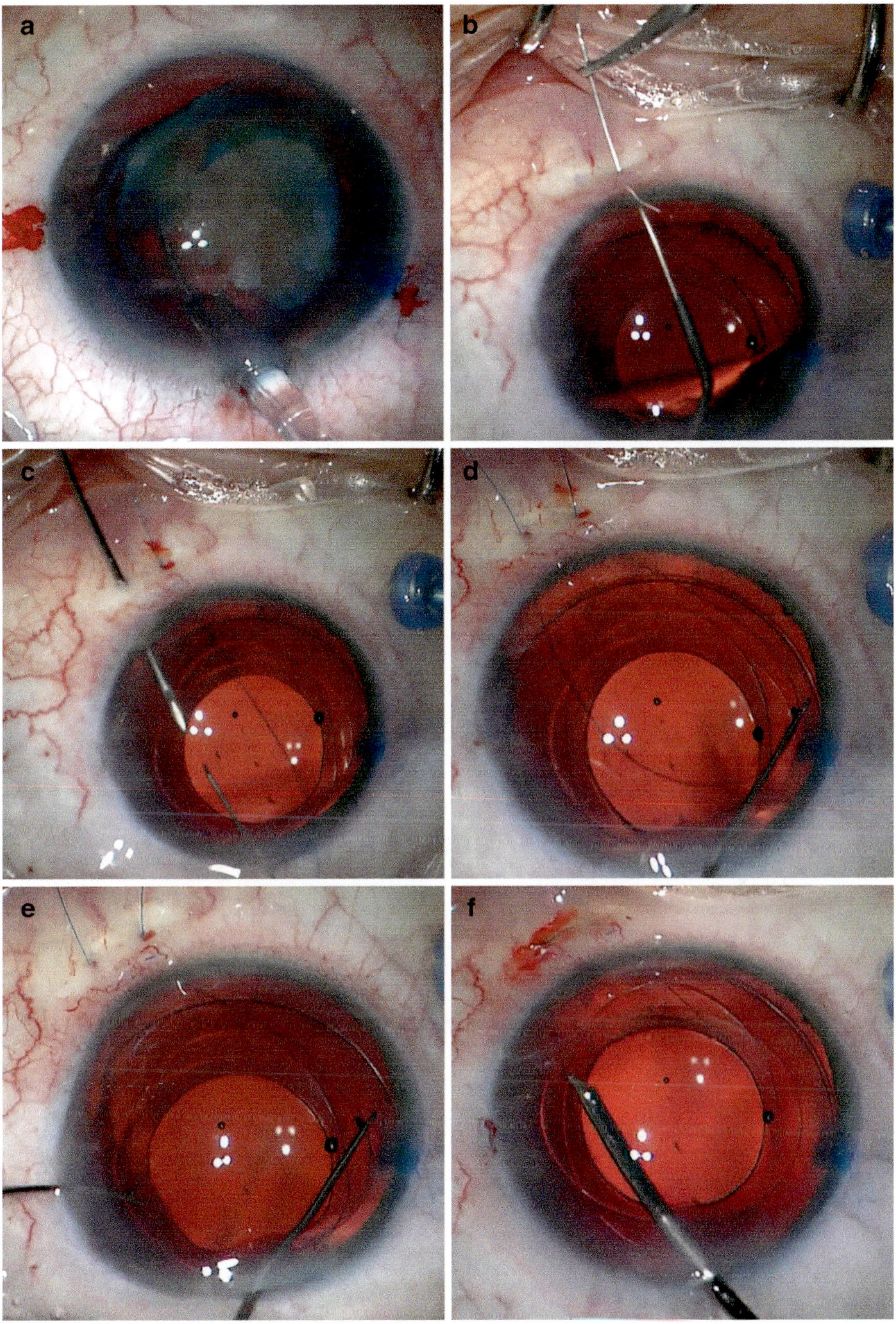

Fig. 17.5 Different steps in the "lasso suture" technique

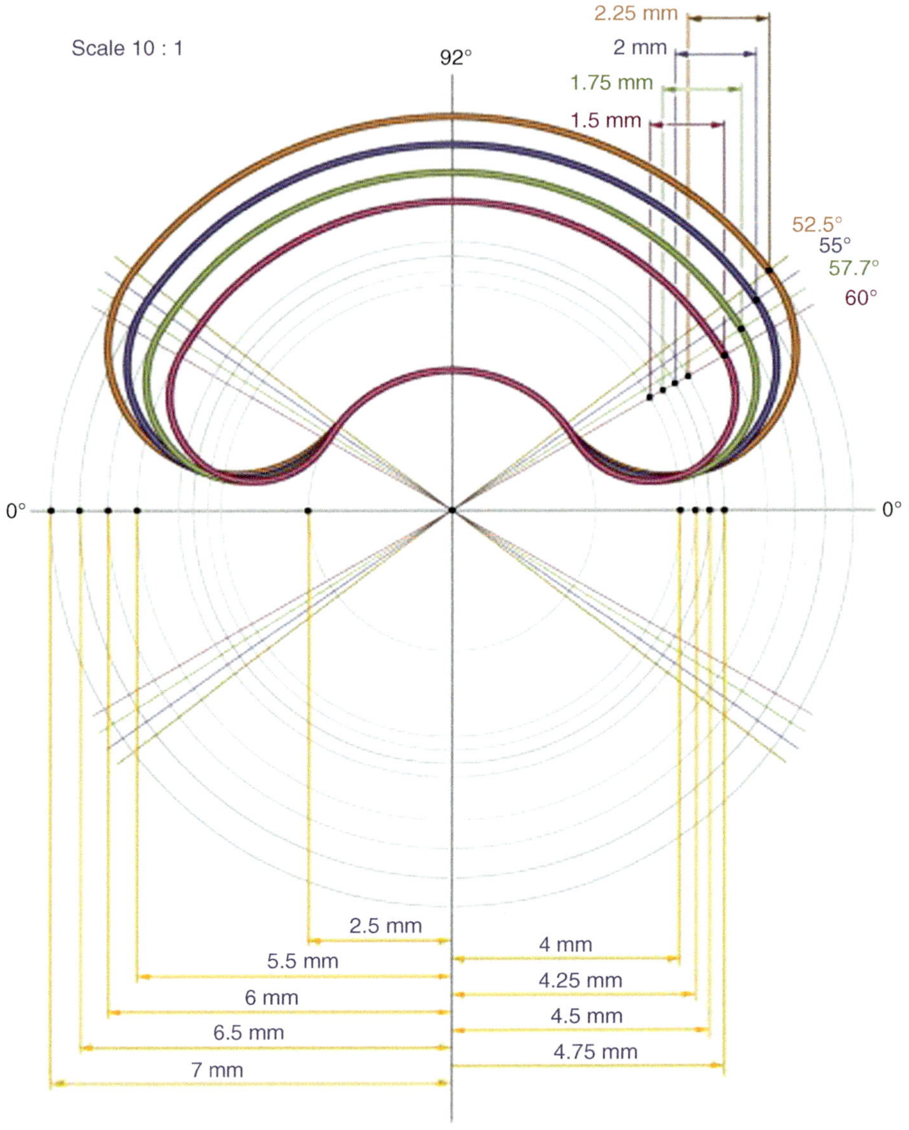

Fig. 17.6 Schematic of the bean-shaped ring segments

The advantage of this device over the "lasso suture" technique is the absence of scleral sutures, probably offering a more permanent solution in younger patients. The bean rings are produced in different outer ring sizes for customized use according to the size of the eye. The inner diameter has a radius of 2.5 mm to fit into the interhaptic groove of the BIL. They should be used in pairs, allowing for 360-degree support. The size of the ring should be calculated by using the white-to-white corneal diameter or by measuring the sulcus diameter with UBM or anterior segment OCT.

17.2.2.1 Surgical Technique

Surgery can be performed under local anaesthesia, but general anaesthesia is preferred in younger patients. A standard approach with two 1.2 mm sideport incisions and a 2.2 mm main incision at the limbus is used. The pupil is dilated with cyclopentolate and phenylephrine preoperatively. OVD is injected into the anterior chamber by using the softshell technique (Viscoat® and Provisc®). In moderate and severe lens luxation, capsulorhexis is better visualized and controlled if the capsule is dyed with Vision Blue®. A small capsulorhexis, preferably not smaller than 3 mm, is made as centrally as possible on the anterior capsule. In cases with mild subluxation, a capsulorhexis of the correct size can be made using a caliper ring no. 5 (Fig. 17.7a). The luxated lens can be centralized with one or more capsular hooks. Thorough hydrodissection will allow nucleus rotation with less force to the remaining zonulas. Careful lens nucleus removal must be done. The cortex is removed with the irrigation-aspiration system taking care not to damage the remaining zonulas. The capsular bag is filled with OVD (Provisc®), and a standard-sized CTR is placed inside the capsular bag (Fig. 17.7b). In more severe cases of zonulolysis, the CTR may have to be placed earlier, during or before lens removal. After nucleus and cortex removal, the guidance ring is placed onto the capsular bag. It is advisable to lift each capsular hook to allow the caliper ring to be placed directly onto the capsule. A cut is made in the existing anterior rhexis, and this is enlarged with the microforceps to the correct size using the caliper ring as a guide. The caliper ring is then removed. The OVD is removed from the capsular bag, and the anterior chamber is filled with it. A small tear is made centrally in the posterior capsule with a 30G needle, and Berger's space is filled with OVD beyond the size of the capsulorhexis. The posterior capsulorhexis is made with a microforceps using the anterior rhexis as guide. If capsular hooks are used, then these can be repositioned through both the anterior and posterior rhexis to support the capsular bag and zonulas during implantation. The main incision is increased to 3.0 mm. The BIL 89A is injected into the anterior chamber and pushed into position close to the capsular bag. The posterior haptic is gently manipulated through both rhexes (Fig. 17.7c). If hooks are used, they should be removed during or after this procedure. After the correct placement of the BIL, the first bean ring is implanted through the main incision and placed in the sulcus (Fig. 17.7d). With a bimanual manoeuvre, the inner ring is placed into the interhaptic grove of the BIL. The same manoeuvre is done with the second bean ring (Fig. 17.7e).

The inner ring of the bean rings should be pushed into the lens groove simultaneously to ensure a correct position. The OVD is removed using the irrigation-aspiration system, and the conjunctiva is closed with Vicryl 8-0 resorbable sutures. Any vitreous in the anterior chamber should be removed using a vitrector. Acetylcholine (Miochol®-E) can be injected to prevent iris capture within the IOL haptics and to test for vitreous prolapse. Cefuroxime (Aprokam®) is installed in the anterior chamber at the end of surgery.

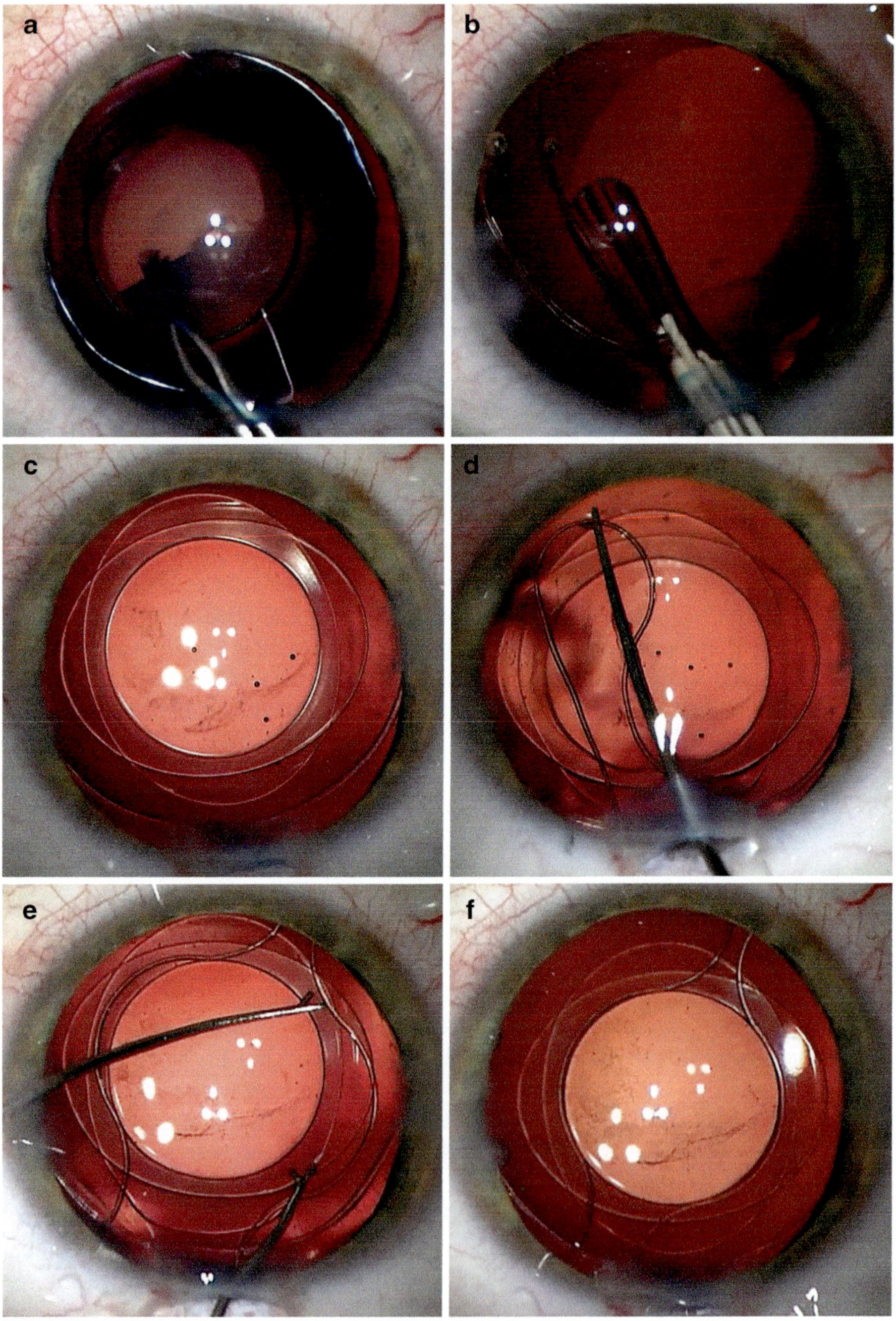

Fig. 17.7 Different steps in the bean ring technique

17.2.2.2 Complications of Bean Rings

- *Iris capture*: When using the bean-shaped rings in the sulcus, the IOL complex is placed slightly more anteriorly, and iris capture and pupillary block are more likely to occur (Fig. 17.8). It is therefore advised to perform an iridectomy peroperatively or a YAG iridotomy pre- or postoperatively. Treatment of iris capture is either medical by dilating the pupil or surgical by repositioning of the BIL. An iridotomy should be made, preventing recapturing by deepening the anterior chamber.
- *Subluxation*: Subluxation of the capsular bag – IOL complex can occur with incorrect placement/dislocation of the bean rings either out of the groove or out of the sulcus. Repositioning or fixation should be considered in these cases. Subluxation can also be the result of bean rings that are too small. In this case, they should be replaced by larger bean rings with greater outer ring diameter or, alternatively, on one side only. Finally, subluxation can occur as a result of asymmetrical anatomy in zonular strength. In this case, consider suturing the IOL complex to the sclera. In some cases, the two bean rings can be sutured together to facilitate better centration.
- *Postoperative refractive challenges*: In cases of zonulolysis, the acceptable postoperative refraction error range is larger than in normal cataract surgery. If unacceptable refractive errors occur, consider contact lens use or corneal surgery as alternatives to lens exchange.

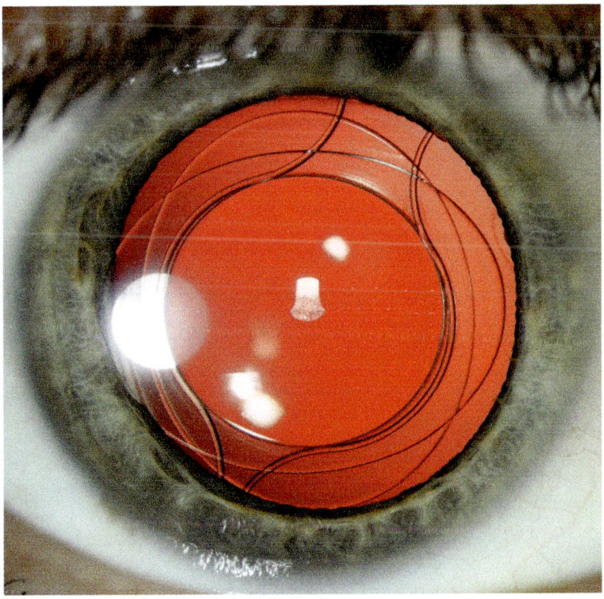

Fig. 17.8 Iris capture after BIL with bean rings, treated by dilating the pupil. Notice the iris captured by the anterior haptic to the left

17.3 Core Messages

- Bag-in-the-lens (BIL) is an excellent option in challenging cases of zonulolysis and lens luxation.
- Instant fixation suture(s) can be placed using "lasso suture" technique, without interfering with the closed capsular bag.
- Remember to empty the capsular bag before performing the posterior rhexis if OVD is used when implanting the CTR.
- The bean rings are suited for sutureless centration of the BIL in younger patients.
- Use a CTR in all cases of zonular weakness.
- Consider iridotomy in cases with bean rings.
- Always have a surgical backup plan.

17.4 Instrument Used

The instruments listed are our preferences, but similar instruments can be used based on the preference of the surgeon.

Item	Description	Manufacturer
Sideport knife	ClearCut 1.2 Dual Bevel	Alcon
Slit knife	ClearCut 2.2 SB	Alcon
OVD	Provisc, Viscoat	Alcon
Hydrodelineator cannula	REF585107	bvi, Visitec
Dye	Vision Blue	DORC
Caliper ring	No. 5	Morcher
Capsulorhexis forceps	K5-090D	Medilens
Capsular tension ring	Eyejet CTR	Morcher
Microforceps	Ikeda angled 30° capsulorhexis 23.0G forceps, Fr2268	EyeTech
Capsular hooks	The Mackool Cataract Support System II (CSSII)	Impex
Suture	Prolene 9-0	Ethicon
Cannula	25G	Braun
Manipulator "Y"	K3-5535	Katena
Forceps Handle 360	Ahmed micrograsper Hoffman/Ahmed horizontal scissors	MST

References

1. Tassignon MJ, Dhubhghaill SN. Bean-shaped ring segments for capsule stretching and centration of bag-in-the-lens cataract surgery. J Cataract Refract Surg. 2014;40:8–12.
2. Simon MA, Origlieri CA, Dinallo AM, Forbes BJ, Wagner RS, Guo S. New management strategies for ectopia lentis. J Pediatr Ophthalmol Strabismus. 2015;52:269–81.
3. Chandra A, Charteris D. Molecular pathogenesis and management strategies of ectopia lentis. Eye. 2014;28:162–8.

4. Christensen AE, Fiskerstrand T, Knappskog PM, Boman H, Rødahl E. A Novel ADAMTSL4 mutation in autosomal recessive ectopia lentis et pupillae. Invest Ophthalmol Vis Sci. 2010;51:6369–73.
5. Hoffman RS, Snyder ME, Devgan U, Allen QB, Yeoh R, Braga-Mele R, For the ASCRS Cataract Clinical Committee, Challenging/Complicated Cataract Surgery Subcommittee. Management of the subluxated crystalline lens. J Cataract Refract Surg. 2013;39:1904–15.
6. Tassignon MJ, Gobin L, Mathysen D, Van Looveren J, De Groot V. Clinical outcomes of cataract surgery after bag-in-the-lens intraocular lens implantation following ISO standard 119797:2006. J Cataract Refract Surg. 2011;37(12):2120–9.

Scleral Anchoring of the Modified Bean-Shaped Ring Segments

18

Anca Cristina Dogaroiu and Sorcha Ní Dhubhghaill

18.1 Introduction

Zonular fibres are suspensory ligaments that hold the lens in its physiological position [1]. These fibres have their origin in the ciliary epithelium and are inserted onto the lens in a circular manner [2]. Defective zonules can be caused by congenital malformations, total or partial agenesis, hereditary metabolic diseases, chronic inflammation and microfibrillopathy and by mechanical disruption [1, 2]. These conditions can be found in pseudoexfoliation syndrome, high myopia, Marfan syndrome, Weill-Marchesani syndrome, ocular trauma or as a result of previous intraocular surgery [1, 2]. The zonular fibres are affected by these pathologies; this causes the zonular weakening or dehiscence and can lead to lens luxation or subluxation. Lens exchange surgery is technically challenging in the presence of lens luxation or subluxation; therefore, this procedure should be performed only by experienced surgeons.

Zonular stabilisation for bag-in-the-lens (BIL) implantation is usually achieved by using bean-shaped ring segments [3]; however, these devices do not offer enough zonular stability when the zonulopathy is severe and, therefore, modified bean-shaped ring segments have been designed in order to facilitate their scleral suturing [4]. Both devices' designs are basically the same; the only difference between them is that the modified bean segments have an eyelet for facilitating scleral suturing (Fig. 18.1) [3].

Electronic Supplementary Material The online version of this chapter (https://doi.org/10.1007/978-3-030-03086-5_18) contains supplementary material, which is available to authorized users.

A. C. Dogaroiu (✉)
ALCOR Ophthalmology Clinic, Bucharest, Romania

S. Ní Dhubhghaill
Department of Ophthalmology, Antwerp University, University Hospital, Edegem, Belgium
e-mail: sorcha.nidhubhghaill@uza.be

M.-J. Tassignon et al. (eds.), *Innovative Implantation Technique*,
https://doi.org/10.1007/978-3-030-03086-5_18

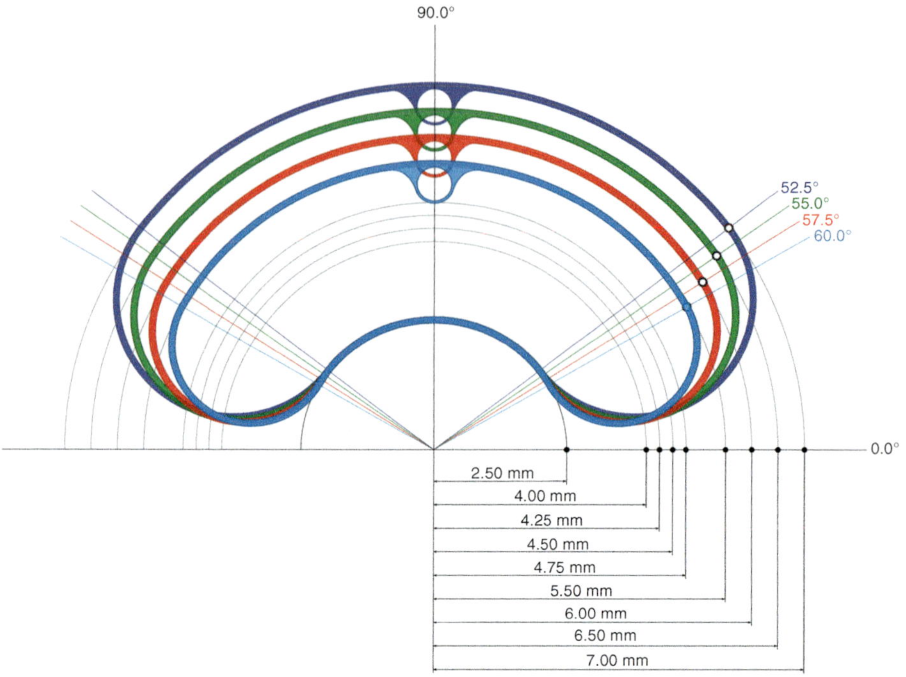

Fig. 18.1 Technical schematic of the modified bean-shaped ring segment

This chapter presents the modified bean-shaped segments' anchoring technique for zonular reinforcement, which is required for bag-in-the-lens (BIL) implantation, by exploring the example of a case of lens-bag complex subluxation [4]. The anchoring technique described in this case could be applied to the special cases mentioned above.

18.2 Indications

The signs of damaged zonules include iridodonesis, phacodonesis, lens subluxation or the presence of vitreous in the anterior chamber [5]. In some of these cases, it is necessary to implant a capsular tension ring – CTR – in order to enhance the lens-bag's stability. These incomplete ring-shaped devices are manufactured from polyethylmethacrylate (PEMA) and have an eyelet at each end [5, 6].

The CTR distributes a centrifugal force towards the capsular bag equator when placed inside the capsular bag, thereby transferring the tension from the area that has intact zonular fibres to areas with zonular weakness or dehiscency [5, 6].

A standard CTR will not offer sufficient support when the zonular dehiscence is greater than four clock hours or in cases of severe zonular laxity. In order to overcome this inconvenience, Cionni has introduced the modified CTR [7] (M-CTR or Cionni ring) which has been specifically designed for scleral anchoring. This is accomplished through a fixation element that is attached to the standard CTR, which ends with an anchoring eyelet [7].

Following Cionni's development, other devices for lens-bag stabilisation have been elaborated, and these include Henderson modified endocapsular tension ring, Ahmed capsular tension segment or the Coloboma shield [5]. Any of these devices could be successfully used in association with the in-the-bag IOL implantation. Unfortunately, these devices could not be used with the bag-in-the-lens (BIL), because their special technique for positioning requires a greater degree of zonular stability [3, 8].

The bean-shaped ring segments were developed on the basis of the standard CTRs [3] and in order to provide additional capsular support, thereby allowing for BIL implantation [8].

The standard bean-shaped ring segments do not provide sufficient support in cases of severe zonular damage, unless they are anchored to sclera; for this reason, an eyelet has been attached to the centre of the inner face of the outer semicircle to facilitate anchoring it to the sclera [4].

18.3 Surgical Technique

A 77-year-old female patient complained of a recent decrease of OD vision. Her ophthalmological history indicated a cataract surgery with CTRs and BIL implantation (+8D lens OD and +3D lens OS) 8 years previously, high myopia bilaterally (OD −13D, OS −14D) and pseudoexfoliation glaucoma. At the time of hospital admission, her best corrected visual acuity was 0.2 (decimal Snellen). The biomicroscope examination of the OD showed an extensive zonular dialysis with lens-bag complex inferior subluxation. In the OS, the biomicroscope examination showed a well-centred BIL and pseudoexfoliative material on the lens surface. A dilated fundus examination revealed OU myopic retinal pigmentary changes and disc excavation secondary to the pseudoexfoliation glaucoma. The autorefractometry for the OD was unmeasurable and was −0.50DS/−1.00 DC @ 173° for the OS. Intraocular pressure was 20 mmHg OD and 19 mm OS with topical medication (latanoprost).

The surgical intervention's first step consisted of a double anaesthesia, both topical with oxybuprocaine and intracameral with both adrenaline (1:1000) and xylocaine solution. After a 3 min isobetadine antiseptic protocol/procedure, the eye was draped with a sterile drape.

A scleral pocket (Fig. 18.2) can be created by using a crescent blade with a starting point in a clear corneal incision in the zonular area that presents maximum dehiscence, according to the scleral fixation technique without the necessity for conjunctival dissection as described by Hoffman et al. [9]. In this way, the need for the following steps can be eliminated: suture knot rotation, sutured wound closure, conjunctival dissection, scleral cauterization and suture [9]. The main incision is made with a blade of 2.8 mm in a clear cornea diametrically opposed to the area of maximum dehiscency. The anterior chamber depth is maintained by intracameral

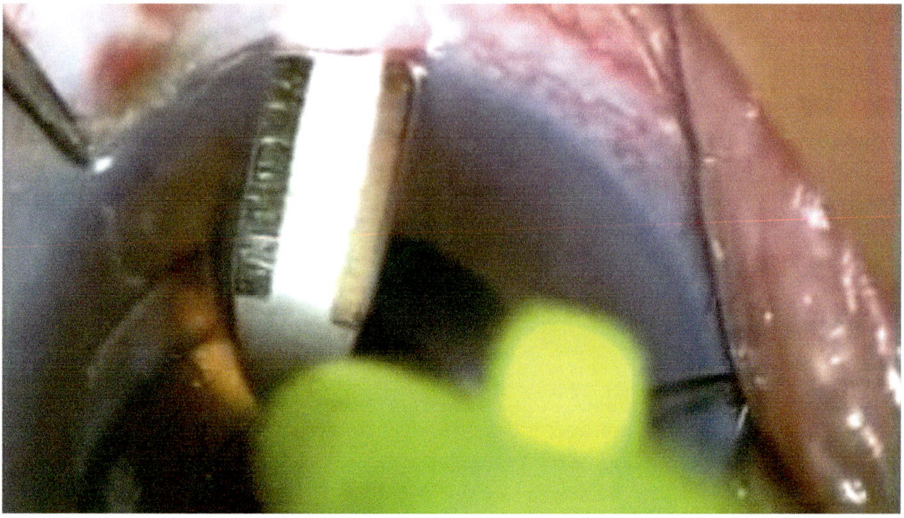

Fig. 18.2 Creation of a Hoffman pocket

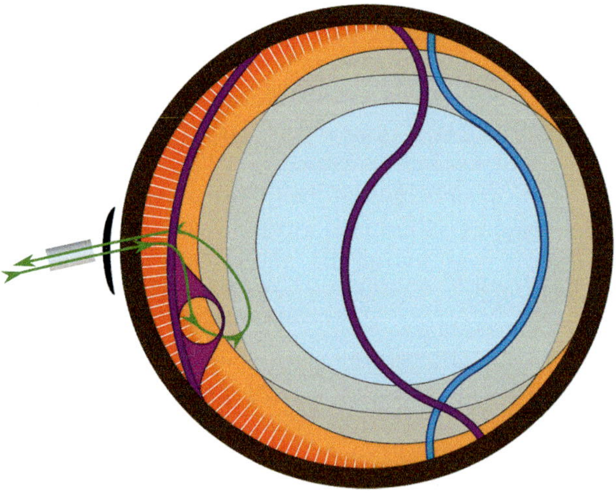

Fig. 18.3 Schematic of the suture bean placement

injections of a cohesive ophthalmic viscosurgical device (OVD) (Healon GV, Abbott Medical Optics).

The modified bean-shaped ring segment is prepared by passing it through its eyelet of a double armed 10-0 Prolene suture twice, on two straight needles with both port needle and forceps.

The two sutures are successively inserted intraocularly through the main incision and externalised parallel to each other at the scleral pocket, approximately 2 mm from the limbus. The bean segment is implanted in the sulcus using a microforceps and is lined up with the scleral pocket by using the secured eyelet (Fig. 18.3). From inside of the scleral pocket, both ends of the 10-0 Prolene suture are retrieved with both a forceps and a microforceps through the limbal corneal incision, located at the scleral pocket base (according to the Hoffman technique), and are tied with two suture-tying forceps [9]. In this way, the knot is protected inside the scleral pocket, thereby eliminating the need for additional scleral and conjunctival sutures.

The scleral anchoring of the modified bean segment permits the insertion of the segment's inner semicircle into the BIL's interhaptic groove [4], by using an instrument with a rounded knob attachment (i.e. Lester manipulator). The implantation of a second modified bean segment is necessary to augment zonular stability.

This second device may or may not be sutured to the sclera in the same way as the first one. The insertion of the second segment inner semicircle into the BIL's interhaptic groove is made by two IOL manipulators, resulting in optimal BIL support and centration [4]. The OVD is washed from the anterior chamber after the lens has been positioned in both modified bean segments.

Carbachol solution is injected into the anterior chamber, as well as cefuroxime (Aprokam®, Thea Pharmaceuticals), to reduce the risk of infection at the end of the surgery as well as to reduce the risk of iris incarceration in the complex formed by the BIL and bean segments.

References

1. American Academy of Ophthalmology. Lens and cataract: section 11, 2014–2015. San Francisco: American Academy of Ophthalmology; 2014.
2. Yanoff M, Duker JS, editors. Ophthalmology. 4th ed. China: Elsevier; 2014.
3. Tassignon MJ, Ní Dhubhghaill S. Bean-shaped ring segments for capsule stretching and centration of bag in the-lens cataract surgery. J Cataract Refract Surg. 2014;40:8 12.
4. Ní Dhubhghaill S, Dogaroiu AC, Zakaria N, Tassignon MJ. Modified bean-shaped ring segments for suture fixation of the bag-in-the-lens intraocular implant. J Cat Refract Surg. 2017;43:1003.
5. Henderson BA, editor. Essentials of cataract surgery. 2nd ed. Thorofare: SLACK Incorporated; 2014.
6. Riedel PJ, Samuelson TW. Capsular tension rings. In: Colvard DM, editor. Achieving excellence in cataract surgery. A step-by-step approach. Self; 2009. p. 115–21.
7. Cionni RJ, Osher RH. Management of profound zonular dialysis or weakness with a new endocapsular ring designed for scleral fixation. J Cataract Refract Surg. 1998;24:1299.
8. Altenburg A, Ní Dhubhghaill SS, Tassignon MJ. Bean-shaped ring segments as a capsule enhancement tool in complex bag in the-Lens intraocular Lens implantation. J Refract Surg. 2017;33(7):454–9.
9. Hoffman RS, Fine IH, Packer M. Scleral fixation without conjunctival dissection. J Cataract Refract Surg. 2006;32:1907–12.

Combined BIL and Vitrectomy

19

Tillmann P. Eckert

Abbreviations

AC	anterior chamber
ACCC	anterior continuous curvilinear capsulorhexis
BIL	“bag in the lens” foldable IOL
BSS	balanced salt solution
CTR	capsular tension ring
HPMC	hydroxypropylmethylcellulose
I/A	irrigation and aspiration
IOFB	intraocular foreign body, -ies
IOL	intraocular lens
OVD	ophthalmic viscoelastic device
PDR	proliferative diabetic retinopathy
PPCCC	primary posterior continuous curvilinear capsulorhexis
PPV	pars plana vitrectomy
PVR	proliferative vitreoretinopathy
RD	retinal detachment

Electronic Supplementary Material The online version of this chapter (https://doi.org/10.1007/978-3-030-03086-5_19) contains supplementary material, which is available to authorized users.

T. P. Eckert (✉)
Eye Clinic, Klinikum Frankfurt Hoechst, Frankfurt am Main, Germany
e-mail: tillmann.eckert@klinikumfrankfurt.de

M.-J. Tassignon et al. (eds.), *Innovative Implantation Technique*,
https://doi.org/10.1007/978-3-030-03086-5_19

19.1 Introduction

Many vitreoretinal surgeons perform simultaneous cataract surgery and vitrectomy, if there is a significant cataract or if a nuclear cataract formation has to be expected soon after a vitrectomy, especially in the presbyopic patient [1].

In complex vitreoretinal diseases (e.g., rhegmatogenous retinal detachments with or without proliferative vitreoretinopathy (PVR), advanced proliferative diabetic retinopathy (PDR) with tractional retinal detachments or in ocular trauma cases with dense vitreous hemorrhages), phacovitrectomy should be considered even in younger patients: The risk of an inadvertent lens touch during vitreous base shaving, dissection and removal of peripheral membranes or laser coagulation of peripheral breaks, and subsequent early cataract formation is quite high. An intraoperative lens opacification can occur during a lengthy operation even without a lens touch and impedes a sufficient visualization of the posterior segment. Removing the crystalline lens and implanting an intraocular lens (IOL) before the vitrectomy enable the surgeon to perform all surgical manipulations, which are necessary for an adequate treatment of the underlying disease, up to the ora serrata and the pars plana.

However, significant fibrinous exudation, posterior synechiae, and early posterior capsular opacification can occur, if cataract and posterior segment surgeries are combined, especially in eyes with a compromised blood-retinal barrier like in PDR, PVR, uveitis, after ocular trauma, or if longer-acting intraocular tamponades are needed [2–7]. An intravitreal gas tamponade can lead to a slight tilt, and decentration of the IOL (even if it was centered perfectly at the end of the surgery, i.e., in the bag with the anterior capsule covering the peripheral optic completely) can result in an early fibrosis of the posterior capsule (Fig. 19.1).

The concept of the "bag in the lens" (BIL) [8] IOL addresses all these potential complications. After a PPCCC and implantation of a BIL, there will be no posterior capsular opacification in the visual axis and no anterior capsule contraction. A YAG capsulotomy is no longer needed in these eyes [9, 10]. The BIL has good long-term stability [11].

Long-acting mydriatics are a risk factor for posterior synechiae after combined surgery [12]. If they are avoided postoperatively, synechiae between the posterior iris and the anterior lens capsule cannot develop because the anterior haptic of the BIL separates the anterior capsule near the capsulorhexis completely from the pupillary margin.

19.2 Methods/Technique

19.2.1 The "Bag in the Lens" Type 89F

In our clinic we started to implant the BIL in 2009. It soon became the IOL of choice for all vitrectomies combined with phacoemulsification and intraocular lens implantation [13].

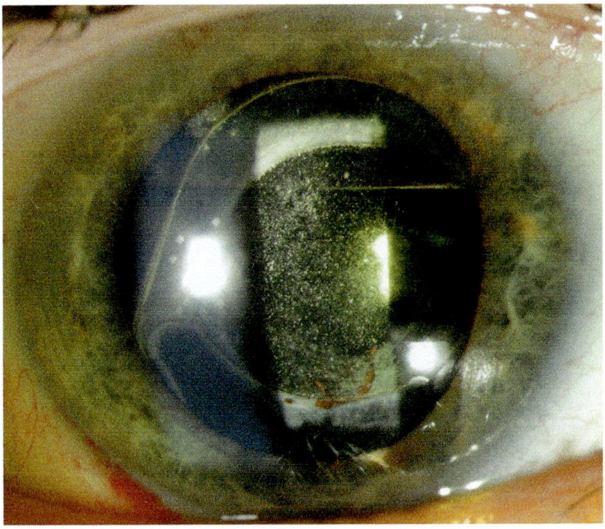

Fig. 19.1 Single-piece IOL with posterior capsular opacification after two vitrectomies for PVR retinal detachment. Inferior haptic in front of anterior capsule

However, starting with the Morcher Type 89A (Morcher, Stuttgart, Germany) which has a diameter of 7.5 mm of both haptics, a pupillary capture occurred in about 38%, mainly in air- or gas-filled in the first postoperative days.

The BIL was modified by enlarging the diameter of the anterior of the two elliptical haptics from 7.5 mm to 8.5 mm (Morcher Type 89F, Fig. 19.2a), while the posterior haptic was not changed (Fig. 19.2b).

The Morcher Type 89F is available from +10 to +30 diopters (on request also from +8.5 to +9.5 diopters) in increments of half diopters. Only in highly myopic patients, the Morcher Type 89A has still to be used (0 diopters to +8.0 diopters in increments of one diopter, on request).

Meanwhile, more than 3000 combined surgeries have been performed in our clinic with the BIL, in the vast majority with Type 89F.

19.2.2 Indications

The BIL can be implanted in every eye undergoing combined phacoemulsification and vitrectomy, if the zonules are stable enough to support an IOL, if an anterior and a primary posterior continuous circular capsulorhexis (ACCC and PPCCC) of an adequate size (between 4.5 and 5.0 mm) have been performed, and if there is no radial tear in the ACCC.

19.2.3 Surgical Technique with the BIL Type 89F

Phacovitrectomy requires peribulbar or general anesthesia. To avoid a positive vitreous pressure, a subsequent retrobulbar or subtenon injection should be postponed

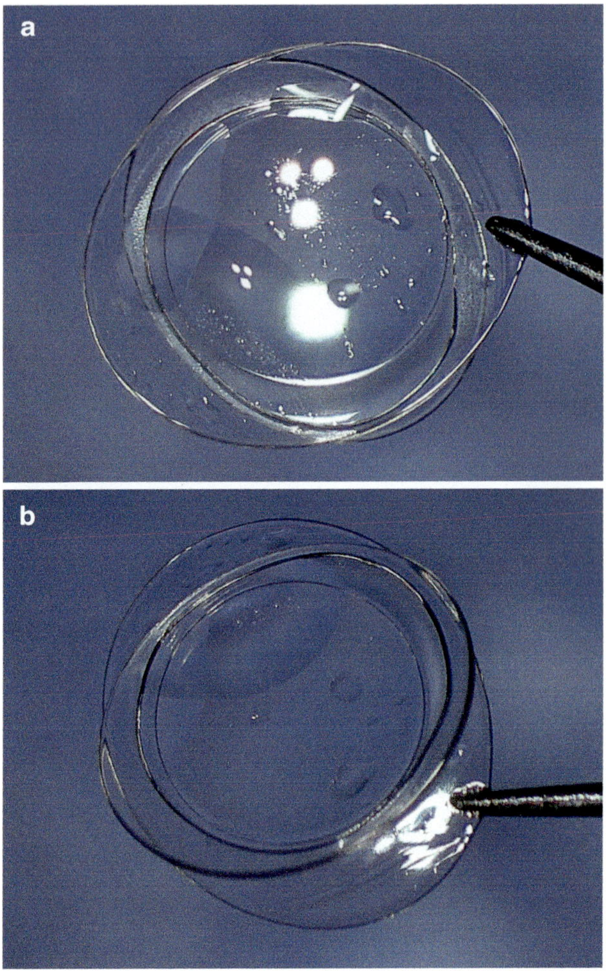

Fig. 19.2 BIL Type 89 F, view from anterior (**a**) and posterior (**b**). The major axis of the elliptical anterior haptic is 8.5 mm and of the posterior haptic only 7.5 mm

until the completion of the PPCCC, if a peribulbar anesthesia fails to produce adequate analgesia and akinesia.

Before starting phacoemulsification, the first pars plana trocar for the infusion line is placed, usually inferotemporally. We use a high flow 27 gauge cannula (DORC, Zuidland, the Netherlands) with the valve left on the cannula. Then a clear corneal incision is performed using a 2.8 mm keratome.

The technique of the anterior continuous circular capsulorhexis (ACCC) is the same as described in Chap. 6: Healon GV (Abbott Medical Optics Inc., Santa Ana, USA) is injected into the anterior chamber (AC), and a 5 mm ring caliper (Morcher) is implanted and centered. An ACCC of 4.5–5.0 mm is carried out within the ring. After hydrodissection and phacoemulsification, the cortex is removed thoroughly with irrigation/aspiration (I/A) and by injection of BSS with a 27 gauge Sauter hydrodissection cannula (Beaver Visitec International, Abingdon, UK) between the peripheral anterior and posterior capsule. Removal of as much of the peripheral cortex remnants as possible is performed to reduce the likelihood of a Soemmerring ring [14] in the future. After flattening the anterior chamber by gentle depression of the posterior lip of the corneal incision, Healon GV is injected with the cannula parallel to iris plane and capsular bag and peripheral to the ACCC. The viscoelastic should not open the capsular bag so that both capsules remain attached to each other.

A PPCCC is much more difficult in a loose posterior capsule. The use of a capsular tension ring (CTR) is recommended if significant folds or wrinkles can be seen in the posterior capsule before puncturing the posterior capsule. A CTR is also used in eyes with pseudoexfoliation, in zonular instability, after ocular trauma, in high myopic eyes, or after a previous vitrectomy. We use an Eyejet CTR type 14 C (Morcher). The CTR can be injected between both capsules without opening the capsular bag with the ophthalmic viscoelastic device (OVD). This is usually possible by simple injection of the CTR into the bag parallel to the plane of the posterior capsule and guiding the ring by gentle movements of the injector.

The PPCCC (see detailed description in Chap. 7) is started with a sharp 30 gauge needle (Becton, Dickinson & Company Ltd., Drogheda, Ireland) mounted on a Healon syringe. It is approached nearly tangential to the central posterior capsule. Immediately before penetration of the posterior capsule, a few radial folds can be seen, which will immediately vanish after penetration of the capsule. After entering Berger's space with the lumen of the needle completely beyond the capsular opening, Healon can be injected slowly in front of the anterior hyaloid without changing instruments. After creating at least a small bubble of Healon behind the posterior capsule, the slit should be enlarged by grasping one edge until a small semicircular flap is created. This helps to prevent a sudden rupture of the posterior capsule while injecting more Healon with the 27 gauge Sauter hydrodissection cannula into Berger's space. The flat cannula can be inserted through one of the two paracentesis to inject Healon behind different parts of the posterior capsular opening. It is very useful to use a high magnification of the operating microscope to be sure that the Healon cannula is directly behind the posterior capsule and not in front of the posterior capsule or behind the anterior hyaloid. The attachments between the anterior hyaloid and the posterior capsule should be completely released beyond the ACCC so that no vitreous can prolapse into the AC. The PPCCC should be slightly smaller or of the same size, but not larger than the ACCC.

We inject the BIL Type 89F through a 3.0 mm corneal incision with the NAVIJECT TM 2.8-1P (LP604410W) injector (Medicel AG, Altenrhein, Switzerland). The BIL has to be laid into the cartridge with the longer anterior haptic upside and with the axis of the anterior haptic parallel to the axis of the injector (Fig. 19.3). Addendum: The NAVIJECT injector is currently not available any more. In our clinic it has been replaced by the Inside® Easy injector 2.4 (O&O mdc Ltd., Lewes, East Sussex, U.K). With this injector a 2.6 mm incision is enough for a wound injection of the BIL Type 89F.

It is important to check the correct entry of the plunger into the cartridge before implanting the IOL under the microscope. A twisted plunger in the cartridge will lead to an increased resistance during the injection of the IOL and can block the complete release of the trailing part of the anterior haptic into the anterior chamber. This could cause a defect of the anterior haptic (Fig. 19.4) we have seen in a few cases.

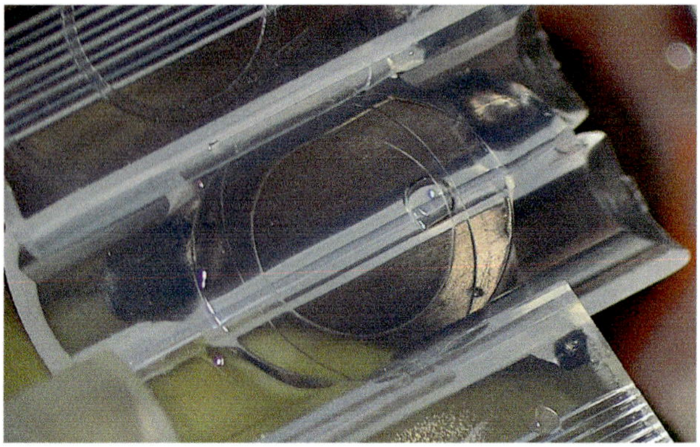

Fig. 19.3 BIL Type 89F in Naviject® cartridge with anterior haptic upside and its major axis parallel to cartridge

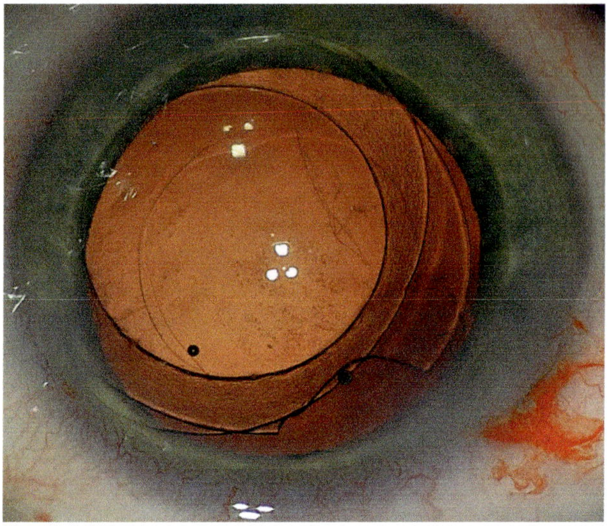

Fig. 19.4 BIL Type 89F with a defect of the anterior haptic after implantation into the AC

The leading haptic should be directed into the space between pupil and anterior capsule. However, the leading haptic can slip inadvertently through the PPCCC into the anterior vitreous cavity. This can be managed by lifting this part of the IOL with a spatula or a cannula (via the corneal tunnel and posterior to the optic) above the capsules (Fig. 19.5).

Usually the trailing haptic remains near the corneal incision after the removal of the injector. With a Healon cannula entering the anterior chamber through the corneal incision or via a paracentesis, this part of the IOL can be pushed down with Healon or the cannula itself. More Healon is injected on top of the optic so that the BIL is parallel to and near the capsules. The implantation is similar to putting a knob into a buttonhole. Starting with one half of the posterior haptic, which is pushed by the Healon cannula or a Neuhann Nucleus Rotator (Geuder AG, Heidelberg, Germany) underneath both capsules, the second half is inserted in

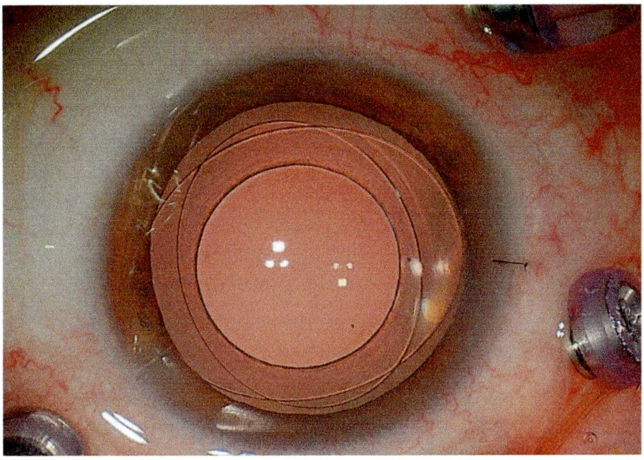

Fig. 19.5 BIL Type 89F after implantation of "bag into lens" in an eye undergoing vitrectomy

small, gentle steps into Berger's space until both capsules are implanted into the groove of the BIL.

If the zonules are weak, a bimanual technique using an iris hook to stretch the rim of ACCC and PPCCC while pushing the second half posterior to the capsules is recommended.

The OVD is removed out of the AC with I/A and a relative low irrigation pressure. With higher irrigation pressures, the AC can be deepened too much which could induce an undesirable constriction of the pupil before the vitrectomy.

The corneal incision is sutured with 10-0 nylon. The suture is usually removed at the end of the surgery.

The other two pars plana trocars (in our clinic usually 23 gauge) are inserted, the infusion line is connected to the inferotemporal trocar, and the vitrectomy is started. The OVD in Berger's space is removed with the vitreous cutter taking care not to engage the posterior capsule.

At the end of the vitrectomy, the pupil is always constricted with Miochol®-E (Bausch + Lomb Incorporated, Rochester, USA). To achieve a sufficient constriction, the injection of adrenaline into the AC should be avoided after the IOL implantation.

19.2.4 Surgical Technique in Eyes with a Reduced or Absent Red Reflex

Cataract surgery in eyes with a markedly reduced or absent reflex can be quite challenging. The ACCC usually can be performed under high magnification of the operating microscope even with no red reflex. Visualization of the anterior capsule during the ACCC or during phacoemulsification can be improved using an intracameral illumination [15–18] (via a sideport incision) or with retroillumination using a chandelier light [19, 20] in the pars plana. The injection of triamcinolone on the anterior capsule [21] or into the anterior vitreous [22] has also been described.

It is important to control the peripheral capsular bag with an endoillumination light probe in the AC since all cortical remnants should be removed before initiation of the PPCCC. After the implantation of the BIL, it is not possible to remove cortical fibers anymore.

If the red reflex is reduced due to a circumscribed preretinal or subretinal hemorrhage, it is sometimes possible to enhance visualization of the posterior capsule by tilting the eye. However, in diabetic patients with a moderate intravitreal and/or preretinal hemorrhage in the beginning of the cataract surgery, the red reflex often deteriorates before starting the PPCCC.

The critical steps of puncturing the posterior capsule, injecting OVD into Berger's space, and starting the PPCCC often require an intracameral illumination. We usually use a shielded 27 gauge illumination probe (DORC) via a paracentesis. A 23 or 25 gauge probe can be used instead through a widened paracentesis or the main incision.

The probe should illuminate the capsular bag tangentially. The posterior capsule is punctured, and Healon is injected carefully through the slit and just behind the posterior capsule (Fig. 19.6).

Reflections of the light on the metallic surfaces of the needle, the forceps, or the Healon cannula can be disturbing. A successful separation of the anterior hyaloid from the posterior capsule can be seen if the blood-stained anterior vitreous moves posteriorly.

If the anterior hyaloid has been perforated too early, the Healon is injected not into Berger's space but into the anterior vitreous. If this happens, it should be attempted to separate the anterior hyaloid from the posterior capsule. Berger's space should be opened with the Healon cannula behind the posterior capsule and in front of the rim of the defect in the anterior hyaloid. Then Healon is injected slowly peripheral to the rim.

An intracameral illumination with a small-gauge endoillumination probe in the paracentesis is also very useful during the implantation of the bag into the IOL (Fig. 19.7).

An alternative approach to intracameral illumination-assisted PPCCC is to improve the red reflex before the PPCCC. The PPV is started to remove the central

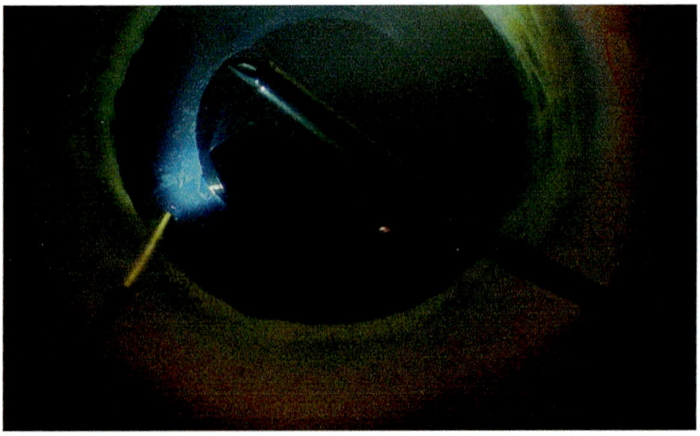

Fig. 19.6 Performing the PCCC in the eye with absent red reflex due to vitreous hemorrhage. Intracameral illumination with a 27 gauge shielded endoillumination probe in paracentesis

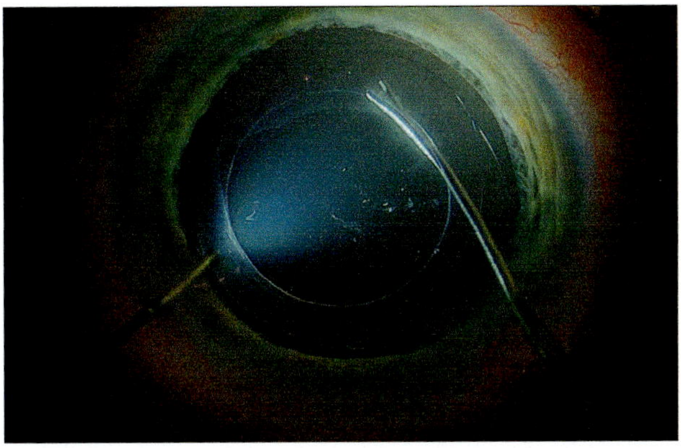

Fig. 19.7 Implantation of the bag into the lens with intracameral illumination (the same eye as in Fig. 19.6)

intravitreal and preretinal hemorrhages but without starting membrane surgery which could cause active bleedings. After having improved the red reflex, it is much easier to identify the anterior hyaloid and to open Berger's space with Healon. A disadvantage of this technique is the increasing mobility of the capsular bag, which tends to have a concave profile after removal of the anterior vitreous. A CTR should be considered. The technique of PPCCC in such a situation is similar to the technique for already vitrectomized eyes described in 19.2.6.

19.2.5 Surgical Technique in Eyes with Posterior Synechiae and/or Small Pupils

If the pupil is too small to perform the ACCC and PCCC safely or if there are posterior synechiae, we use five iris retractors (Alcon/Grieshaber) to dilate the pupil to about 5–5.5 mm, so that the caliper ring can be seen completely. After the BIL is implanted, the iris hooks are removed, and the corneal incision is sutured. The viscoelastic is left in the AC to avoid flattening of the AC and pupillary constriction. Usually, the pupil remains wide enough to reach the peripheral retina and the vitreous base by indentation. Before the last fluid-air exchange and the injection of the tamponading agent, the OVD is removed from the AC with bimanual I/A. Postoperative mydriatics are not necessary since posterior synechiae will not develop again even after heavy fibrin exudation in the first days. Fibrinous membranes are only treated with hourly local steroids.

19.2.6 Surgical Technique in Vitrectomized Eyes

If a phakic eye has been already vitrectomized, cataract surgery can be difficult, especially in myopic eyes with a deep chamber and in eyes with decreased zonular stability. Even with lower irrigation pressures, the anterior chamber can be very deep during phacoemulsification, and the pupil tends to constrict early.

A CTR should be implanted to stabilize the posterior capsule. However, the absence of significant amounts of vitreous behind the posterior capsule makes it more flaccid. Puncturing such a posterior capsule is more difficult than in a non-vitrectomized eye and should be carried out only with a sharp needle.

Healon injected into Berger's space can separate even a thin layer of anterior hyaloid, but often the viscoelastic simply falls into the vitreous cavity.

Because there is no barrier between posterior segment and anterior chamber, the eye can become too soft.

Therefore, the pars plana infusion should be connected to the first trocar before starting the PCCC. Irrigation pressures should be set to low values (5 mm Hg). By intermittent activation of the infusion, one can pressurize the vitreous cavity with small amounts of fluid as needed. Higher irrigation pressures could press the OVD out of the AC via the corneal incision and should be avoided. Using this technique, it is usually possible to perform the PPCCC.

Because of the increased elasticity of the posterior capsule, a smaller opening should be attempted by pulling the posterior capsule more to the center than usual (similar to an ACCC in children). Implanting the capsular bag into the groove of the BIL is easier after closure of the corneal incision with the OVD still in the AC. With the pars plana infusion on, the posterior haptic is positioned behind the PCCC using a Neuhann Nucleus Rotator or a similar instrument through a paracentesis. The OVD can be removed with bimanual I/A after successful implantation of the BIL.

19.2.7 Surgical Technique in Gas-Filled Eyes

If an early reoperation in a phakic eye is necessary, and there is still air or gas in the eye, this should be removed via the pars plana before starting the PCCC. All three trocars should be inserted before starting the PCCC.

Small air or gas bubbles behind the posterior capsule can be tolerated since they can be displaced by injection of Healon or by removing them via the AC.

19.2.8 Surgical Technique in Silicone Oil-Filled Eyes

The buoyancy of silicone oil leads to a convex contour of the capsular bag after removal of the lens cortex. This improves the apposition of both capsules and facilitates the PPCCC compared to vitrectomized eyes without oil tamponade. Therefore, it is not useful to remove the oil before the PPCCC. After filling the AC with Healon GV as usual, implanting a CTR and puncturing the posterior capsule, the oil can be separated easily from the posterior capsule with Healon. If this is accomplished, no silicone oil will prolapse into the AC during the PPCCC.

Theoretically, it would be possible to aspirate the silicone oil through the PPCCC [24–27]. We prefer to remove the silicone oil after implantation of the BIL with active aspiration through one of the 23 gauge pars plana cannulas to protect the corneal endothelium.

19.3 Special Indications

19.3.1 Posterior Capsule Rupture

In a complicated cataract surgery with a rupture of the posterior capsule, the BIL is an alternative to a sulcus-fixated IOL, if the ACCC is intact and not larger than 5.0 mm. After anterior vitrectomy, the anterior (if too small) and the posterior capsular opening are enlarged (if smaller than the ACCC) with microscissors and an end-gripping microforceps to a size of 4.5–5.0 mm.

This is also true for all combined phacovitrectomies with an inadvertent posterior capsule rupture.

19.3.2 Penetrating Ocular Trauma

In penetrating traumas with a perforation of the crystalline lens peripheral to the central 7 mm a normal 5 mm, ACCC is usually possible. After the removal of the nucleus and cortex, the posterior capsule defect often extends into the center of the posterior capsule. After vitrectomy of the anterior vitreous, such a defect can be converted into a noncontinuous posterior capsulorhexis of about 5 mm with small-gauge microscissors and microforceps through the pars plana cannulas or through a paracentesis. Then the ACCC and at least parts of the posterior capsule can be implanted into the groove of the BIL leading to an acceptable stability.

19.3.3 IOFB Removal Through PPCCC

Intravitreal foreign bodies (IOFB) of appropriate size can be removed through the capsular openings with an endomagnet or with microforceps pulling or grasping the IOFB out of the anterior vitreous cavity, if they fit through the corneal incision [28–30]. The corneal endothelium should be protected by OVD. During the extraction through the AC the infusion is deactivated. The lens is implanted afterward.

19.3.4 Uveitis

Especially in inflamed eyes and in chronic uveitis, the BIL is a very good option. A synechiolysis and pupillary dilation with iris hooks are often needed.

Posterior synechiae cannot arise, even after a heavy postoperative fibrin exudation, because the paracentral and mid peripheral anterior capsule is covered by the anterior haptic. Aggressive steroid treatment should be applied in the first week. Surprisingly, these eyes calm down rather quickly. Giant cells on the hydrophilic IOL can be found postoperatively, especially in chronic uveitis or advanced PDR. Usually this reaction is relatively mild.

19.4 Complications Related to the IOL Design

19.4.1 Condensation on the Posterior Surface of the BIL During Fluid-Air Exchange

After a fluid-air exchange, condensating water vapor will almost always cover the posterior surface of the hydrophilic BIL at least in parts and deteriorates the view on the fundus significantly. If further intravitreal manipulations under air are necessary (e.g., drainage of subretinal fluid, laser coagulation of breaks, peripheral vitrectomy), this can be very annoying (Fig. 19.8).

One drop of hydroxypropylmethylcellulose (HPMC) 2% (e.g., Aurovisc®, Aurolab, Madurai, India) applied on the posterior surface of the BIL eliminates the condensation completely and restores a good visualization of the retina.

19.4.2 Pupillary Capture

A pupillary or iris capture is a known complication of the BIL, even in normal cataract surgery [8, 10]. It can occur also with other IOL types, if the optic is not covered completely by the capsular bag (e.g., in sulcus-fixated IOL). In a retrospective analysis of combined cataract extraction and pars plana vitrectomy, 1-piece IOLs "in the bag" were more prone to pupillary capture than 3-piece IOLs [23].

Pupillary capture is the most common BIL-related complication in combined phacovitrectomy (about 7% in our series). The likelihood of a pupillary capture is higher in gas-filled eyes. This is also true after reoperations in an eye with a BIL.

The intravitreal gas bubble can tilt the BIL and push one or even both haptics in front of the pupillary plane, especially if the patients lie in a supine position, for

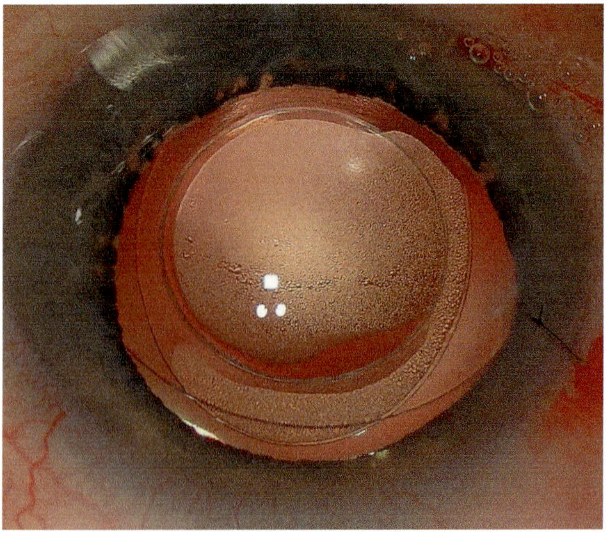

Fig. 19.8 Condensation of water vapor on posterior surface of BIL immediately after an fluid-air exchange

example, in the postanesthesia recovery. When the pupil is constricting during this period, parts of the iris can get caught into the groove of the BIL. In most of the cases, three to six clock hours of incarceration are found, usually in the first postoperative days. With a longer-acting gas such as C2F6, a pupillary capture can occur even after the first week.

To prevent a pupillary capture, Miochol®-E is injected at the end of surgery to constrict the pupil. Even small intracameral doses of acetylcholine can induce a bradycardia and hypotension. Therefore, the anesthetist should always be informed if intracameral Miochol®-E is used. Blood pressure and heart rate should be monitored in the first hour after the intracameral injection. In our clinic every patient receives 0.25 mg intravenous atropine prophylactically at the end of the surgery.

Even a slight leakage through one of the corneal incisions at the end of the operation should not be tolerated since a flat AC favors a pupillary capture. If the pupil remains relatively wide, it should be checked that the anterior haptics are behind the pupil.

The patient is advised to avoid a supine position. Mydriatics must not be applied postoperatively as long as a significant amount of gas is in the eye (about 3 days in an eye with a complete air fill, about 1 week using SF6 and even more with a longer-acting gas like C2F6). Usually it is possible to see the peripheral retina in a gas-filled eye without dilating the pupil.

However, at the end of the vitrectomy, some pupils cannot be constricted sufficiently or the patient lies on his back, or mydriatics are applied too early or inadvertently.

If there is only a partial pupillary capture, repeated application of short-acting mydriatics can lead to a complete dilation of the iris pulling the pupillary margin out of the groove of the BIL. The patient should be asked to maintain a prone position for the following hours in order to minimize the pressure of the intravitreal gas on the BIL. With continued prone positioning, the pupil can constrict in front of the BIL within the next hours (Fig. 19.9).

In most cases we prefer to reposition the incarcerated iris. A slim iris spatula is put through a paracentesis opposite to the captured area into the AC and underneath

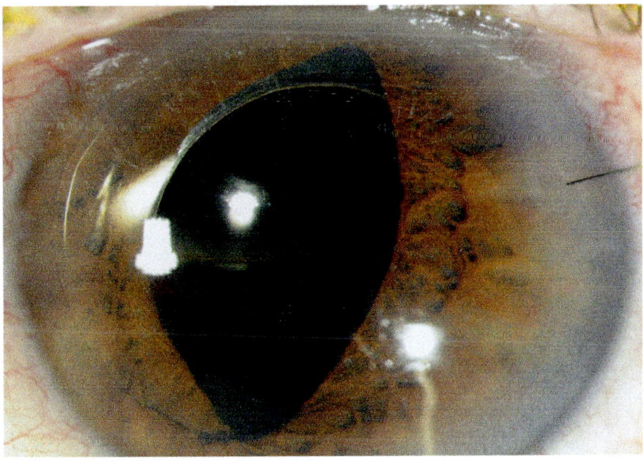

Fig. 19.9 Partial pupillary capture on the second day after phacovitrectomy with air tamponade

the pupil near the captured part. With a sliding motion of the spatula parallel to and in front of the BIL, the captured iris is pulled out of the groove of the BIL. This should be done in the operating room under topical or intracameral anesthesia.

Trying to push the haptic in front of the iris behind the pupil should not be intended, since this can lead to a luxation of the BIL into the vitreous cavity.

In the rare event of a complete pupillary capture during the first postoperative days, there is a risk of pupillary block glaucoma. This situation requires a bimanual technique using two spatulas. The tip of the first iris spatula is inserted tangentially into the groove near the incarcerated area then behind the incarcerated iris. While pushing the pupillary margin to the periphery, the second spatula engages the pupil from a paracentesis opposite to the first spatula. This second iris spatula is sliding under the pupil until the first half of the haptic is covered with the iris again. The second half of the pupil can be repositioned as described. In a gas-filled eye, it is much easier to perform this maneuver after having filled the AC with an OVD. This is removed bimanually after repositioning the iris.

19.5 Silicone Oil

Silicone oil can be used in combination with the BIL without any restrictions. The silicone oil can be removed completely from the optic. However, numerous small emulsified oil droplets can get caught into the groove of the BIL which can be seen under high magnification (Fig. 19.10). These droplets cannot be removed by irrigation or aspiration.

19.6 Troubleshooting

If vitreous enters the AC before implantation, remove the vitreous with the vitreous cutter through the pars plana cannulas first. If needed, triamcinolone acetonide can be injected into the AC to enhance a complete removal of vitreous strands in the AC and near the lens capsule. Only implant the BIL after complete removal of the anterior vitreous.

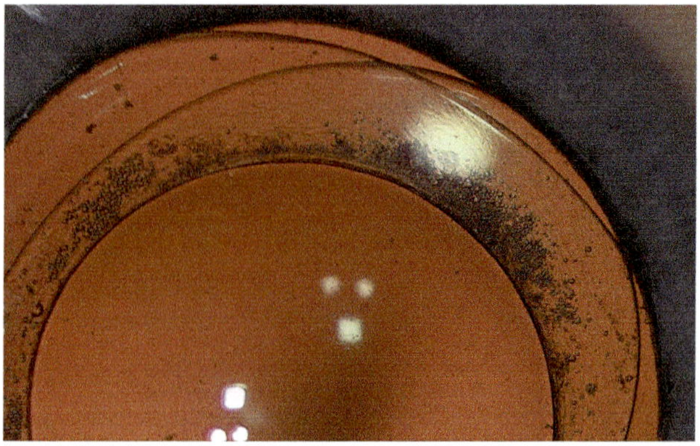

Fig. 19.10 Retained emulsified oil droplets in the groove of the BIL after silicone oil removal

19.7 Disadvantages of Combined BIL and Vitrectomy Compared to Phacovitrectomy with a Standard IOL

To date the price for the BIL is higher than for a standard IOL. In addition a ring caliper and the second OVD are needed. The IOL can be ordered only after an instructional course [31]. There is a learning curve. The cataract surgery (mainly the PPCCC) takes at least a few minutes longer. The PPCCC can be quite difficult, especially in eyes with a reduced or absent red reflex. In air- or gas-filled eyes, a diagnostic mydriasis has to be avoided in the first postoperative days. Pupillary capture can occur also in reoperations requiring an air or a gas tamponade.

19.8 Core Messages About the BIL in Vitreoretinal Surgery

The "bag in the lens" (BIL) IOL can be used in every vitreoretinal disease requiring phacovitrectomy, even in complex and advanced diseases.

The BIL offers a good intraoperative and postoperative visualization up to the peripheral retina and an excellent intraoperative stability, also during scleral indentation.

A posterior capsular opacification and a contraction of the anterior capsule can be avoided completely. In most cases the capsular bag remains relatively transparent. A postoperative YAG capsulotomy is not necessary anymore.

Until now we haven't seen an opacification of the surface of the hydrophilic IOL [32], although most IOLs were in contact with air or gas.

If ACCC and PPCCC are of appropriate size, there will be no postoperative decentration of the BIL, even after a gas tamponade.

The AC becomes quiet within a few days, even in eyes with fibrinous exudation.

Outstanding is that even eyes with acute or chronic inflammation will never develop posterior synechiae or a seclusio pupillae. The pupil always remains mobile. This is especially helpful in eyes requiring further surgeries.

In posterior capsule defects, the BIL can be used as a backup lens instead of a sulcus-fixated IOL, if the ACCC has remained intact and is not wider than 5 mm.

If an exchange of the BIL is needed (e.g., after false biometry in macular-off RD), a BIL is much easier to explant [33] than a conventional single-piece or three-piece IOL out of a fibrotic capsular bag.

Pupillary capture can be avoided in most cases by using the Morcher Type 89F, constricting the pupil with acetylcholine at the end of the vitrectomy and by avoiding mydriatics in the first postoperative days.

19.9 Instruments/Tools Used During Combined BIL and Vitrectomy

This is a personal selection. Similar instruments can be used instead.

Item	Product (number)	Manufacturer
"Bag in the lens" foldable IOL	Type 89F: 8.5–30 dpt. Type 89A: 0–8 dpt.	Morcher, Stuttgart, Germany
Ring caliper	Ring Caliper Type 5	Morcher
Capsular tension ring	Eyejet CTR type 14C (PMMA 11–13 mm)	Morcher
Lens injection system	Naviject® Injector Set 2.8 mm (LP604410W) Addendum: Inside® Easy injector 2.4	Medicel AG, Altenrhein, Switzerland Addendum: O&O mdc Ltd., Lewes, East Sussex, UK
OVD	Healon Healon GV	Abbott Medical Optics, Santa Ana, USA
Capsulorhexis forceps	Mohr Capsulorhexis Forceps (50.265)	DORC International, Zuidland, the Netherlands
23 gauge microforceps	Eckardt End-gripping (1286.W06)	DORC International
23 gauge microscissors	Straight (1286.J06) Curved Horizontal (1286.M06)	DORC International
23 gauge light fiber	Eckardt Multi-Fiber Endoillumination Probe/ Chandelier (3269.MF06)	DORC International
27 gauge light fiber	Shielded Totalview Endoillumination Probe (3269.SBS04)	DORC International
30 gauge cannula	BD Microlance 3 30 Gauge 1/2 inch (304000)	Becton, Dickinson & Company Ltd., Drogheda, Ireland
Hydrodissection cannula	Sauter 27 gauge Flat Tip Nucleus Hydrodissector (585099)	Beaver Visitec International, Abingdon, UK
Nucleus rotator	Thomas Neuhann Nucleus Rotator (G-32160)	Geuder AG
Iris hook	Frankfurt Model Iris Hook and Lens Manipulator (G-31911)	Geuder AG
Iris retractors	Flexible Iris Retractor (611.74)	Alcon / Grieshaber AG, Schaffhausen, Switzerland
Balanced salt solution	BSS®	Alcon, Fort Worth, USA
Acetylcholine chloride 10 mg/ml	Miochol®-E	Bausch + Lomb Incorporated, Rochester, USA
Hydroxypropylmethylcellulose (HPMC) 2%	Aurovisc® Hypromellose Ophthalmic Solution 2%	Aurolab, Madurai, India

Financial Disclosure The author has no financial interest in any material or method mentioned.

References

1. Steel DHW. Phacovitrectomy: expanding indications. J Cataract Refract Surg. 2007;33(6):933–6. https://doi.org/10.1016/j.jcrs.2007.01.047.
2. Ebihara Y, Kato S, Oshika T, et al. Posterior capsule opacification after cataract surgery in patients with diabetes mellitus. J Cataract Refract Surg. 2006;32(7):1184–7. https://doi.org/10.1016/j.jcrs.2006.01.100.
3. Kim S-W, Oh J, Song J-S, et al. Risk factors of iris posterior synechia formation after phacovitrectomy with three-piece acrylic IOL or single-piece acrylic IOL. Ophthalmologica. 2009;223(4):222–7. https://doi.org/10.1159/000203366.
4. Makhzoum O, Crosby NJ, Hero M. Secondary angle-closure glaucoma due to posterior synechiae formation following phacovitrectomy. Int Ophthalmol. 2011;31(6):481–2. https://doi.org/10.1007/s10792-011-9475-3.
5. Park SP, Ahn JK, Lee GH. Morphologic changes in the anterior segment after phacovitrectomy for proliferative diabetic retinopathy. J Cataract Refract Surg. 2009;35(5):868–73. https://doi.org/10.1016/j.jcrs.2008.12.032.
6. Roh JH, Sohn HJ, Lee DY, et al. Comparison of posterior capsular opacification between a combined procedure and a sequential procedure of pars plana vitrectomy and cataract surgery. Ophthalmologica. 2010;224(1):42–6. https://doi.org/10.1159/000234907.
7. Toda J, Kato S, Oshika T, et al. Posterior capsule opacification after combined cataract surgery and vitrectomy. J Cataract Refract Surg. 2007;33(1):104–7. https://doi.org/10.1016/j.jcrs.2006.09.018.
8. Tassignon M-JB, de GV, Vrensen GF. Bag-in-the-lens implantation of intraocular lenses. J Cataract Refract Surg. 2002;28(7):1182–8. https://doi.org/10.1016/S0886-3350(02)01375-5.
9. Leysen I, Coeckelbergh T, Gobin L, et al. Cumulative neodymium: YAG laser rates after bag-in-the-lens and lens-in-the-bag intraocular lens implantation: comparative study. J Cataract Refract Surg. 2006;32(12):2085–90. https://doi.org/10.1016/j.jcrs.2006.07.025.
10. Tassignon M-J, Gobin L, Mathysen D, et al. Clinical outcomes of cataract surgery after bag-in-the-lens intraocular lens implantation following ISO standard 11979-7:2006. J Cataract Refract Surg. 2011;37(12):2120–9. https://doi.org/10.1016/j.jcrs.2011.06.025.
11. Verbruggen KHM, Rozema JJ, Gobin L, et al. Intraocular lens centration and visual outcomes after bag-in-the-lens implantation. J Cataract Refract Surg. 2007;33(7):1267–72. https://doi.org/10.1016/j.jcrs.2007.03.022.
12. Lee SB, Lee DG, Kwag JY, et al. The effect of mydriatics on posterior synechia after combined pars plana vitrectomy, phacoemulsification, and intraocular lens implantation. Retina. 2009;29(8):1150–4. https://doi.org/10.1097/IAE.0b013e3181a3b85c.
13. Eckardt C. Combined phacovitrectomy Retina Today. 2013. (5/6):36–38.
14. Werner L, Tassignon M-J, Zaugg BE, et al. Clinical and histopathologic evaluation of six human eyes implanted with the bag-in-the-lens. Ophthalmology. 2010;117(1):55–62. https://doi.org/10.1016/j.ophtha.2009.06.031.
15. Jung Y, Kim IN, Yoon J, et al. Intracameral illuminator-assisted advanced cataract surgery combined with 23-gauge vitrectomy in eyes with poor red reflex. J Cataract Refract Surg. 2013;39(6):845–50. https://doi.org/10.1016/j.jcrs.2012.12.036.
16. Kim K-H, Sohn HJ, Song HJ, et al. Surgeon-controlled-endoillumination-guided irrigation and aspiration during combined 23-gauge sutureless vitrectomy and cataract surgery in eyes with poor fundus reflex. J Cataract Refract Surg. 2010;36(12):2028–31. https://doi.org/10.1016/j.jcrs.2010.10.004.
17. Park YM, Park JY, Lee JS, et al. Comparative analysis of brilliant blue G and an intracameral illuminator in assisting visualization of the anterior capsule in eyes with vitreous hemorrhage. J Cataract Refract Surg. 2016;42(7):1015–21. https://doi.org/10.1016/j.jcrs.2016.03.038.
18. Yamamoto N, Ozaki N, Murakami K. Trypan-blue- and endoillumination-assisted phacoemulsification in eyes with vitreous hemorrhage during combined cataract and vitreous surgery. Ophthalmologica. 2005;219(6):338–44. https://doi.org/10.1159/000088375.

19. Bilgin S, Kayikcioglu O. Chandelier retroillumination-assisted cataract surgery during vitrectomy. Eye (Lond). 2016;30(8):1123–5. https://doi.org/10.1038/eye.2016.112.
20. Jang SY, Choi KS, Lee SJ. Chandelier retroillumination-assisted cataract extraction in eyes with vitreous hemorrhage. Arch Ophthalmol. 2010;128(7):911–4. https://doi.org/10.1001/archophthalmol.2010.120.
21. Furino C, Alessio G, Recchimurzo N, et al. Anterior capsule staining using micronized triamcinolone in the absence of red reflex. J Cataract Refract Surg. 2011;37(6):983–6. https://doi.org/10.1016/j.jcrs.2011.03.028.
22. Tanikawa A, Horiguchi M. Intravitreal triamcinolone-illuminated cataract surgery for patients with dense vitreous hemorrhage. JAMA Ophthalmol. 2015;133(1):93–4. https://doi.org/10.1001/jamaophthalmol.2014.3321.
23. Rudnisky CJ, Cheung J, Nanji JA. Intraocular lens capture in combined cataract extraction and pars plana vitrectomy: Comparison of 1-piece and 3-piece acrylic intraocular lenses. J Cataract Refract Surg. 2010;36(10):1645–9. https://doi.org/10.1016/j.jcrs.2010.04.037.
24. Avci R. Cataract surgery and transpupillary silicone oil removal through a single scleral tunnel incision under topical anesthesia; sutureless surgery. Int Ophthalmol. 2001;24(6):337–41.
25. Boscia F, Recchimurzo N, Cardascia N, et al. Phacoemulsification with transpupillary silicone oil removal and lens implantation through a corneal incision using topical anesthesia. J Cataract Refract Surg. 2003;29(6):1113–9.
26. Dada VK, Talwar D, Sharma N, et al. Phacoemulsification combined with silicone oil removal through a posterior capsulorhexis. J Cataract Refract Surg. 2001;27(8):1243–7.
27. Loncar VL, Petric I, Vatavuk Z, et al. Phacoemulsification and silicone oil removal through the planned posterior capsulorhexis. Coll Antropol. 2005;29(Suppl 1):63–6.
28. Boiko EV, Churashov SV, Kulikov AN, et al. Clear corneal phacovitrectomy with posterior capsulorhexis and IOL implantation in management of selective vitreoretinal cases. J Ophthalmol. 2015;2015:474072. https://doi.org/10.1155/2015/474072.
29. Kunikata H, Uematsu M, Nakazawa T, et al. Successful removal of large intraocular foreign body by 25-gauge microincision vitrectomy surgery. J Ophthalmol. 2011;2011:940323. https://doi.org/10.1155/2011/940323.
30. Park JH, Lee JH, Shin JP, et al. Intraocular foreign body removal by viscoelastic capture using DisCoVisc during 23-gauge microincision vitrectomy surgery. Retina. 2013;33(5):1070–2. https://doi.org/10.1097/IAE.0b013e318286ce83.
31. MORCHER® GmbH (2012) Bag-in-the-lens. IOL and Technique. http://www.morcher.com/fileadmin/content/Broschueren_Kataloge/CATALOG-89A-TASSIGNON_2012-05-02.pdf. Accessed 28 May 2017.
32. Walker NJ, Saldanha MJ, Sharp JAH, et al. Calcification of hydrophilic acrylic intraocular lenses in combined phacovitrectomy surgery. J Cataract Refract Surg. 2010;36(8):1427–31. https://doi.org/10.1016/j.jcrs.2010.04.011.
33. Ni Dhubhghaill S, van Os L, de Keizer RJW, et al. Intraocular lens exchange technique for an opacified bag-in-the-lens. J Cataract Refract Surg. 2015;41(5):924–8. https://doi.org/10.1016/j.jcrs.2015.04.006.

IOL Dislocation and the Diving BIL

20

Ernesto Bali, Haroon Haider, and Marie-José Tassignon

20.1 Introduction

Since Harold Ridley, rehabilitation after cataract surgery has been revolutionized by the implantation of an IOL. The IOL restores, and often improves, the focus of light rays upon the retina. Unfortunately, Ridley's lens design was abandoned due to the nearly 10% dislocation rate. Improvements in surgical technique, lens material and lens design decreased the likelihood of postoperative IOL malposition ever since. The incidence of malpositioned IOLs still remains significant but is not the major cause for patient dissatisfaction. Incorrect lens power has become the leading reason for IOL explantation in recent years.

20.2 Classification and Aetiology of Lens Dislocations

IOL malpositioning can be divided into three categories:

1. Dislocation (luxation), consisting of the complete loss of the lens into the vitreous cavity due to zonular lysis or IOL implantation in an unsecure capsular bag. It occurs with an incidence of 0.8–1.2% [1, 2].
2. Clinically significant decentration (subluxation), due to capsule contraction or zonular lysis. In this case part of the lens remains in the posterior chamber. Its incidence is about 3% [2].

E. Bali (✉)
Delta Hospital CHIREC group, Brussels, Belgium
e-mail: ernesto.bali@chirec.be

H. Haider
Delta Hospital CHIREC group, Brussels, Belgium

Department of Medicine and allied sciences, Antwerp University, Wilrijk, Belgium

M.-J. Tassignon
Department of Ophthalmology, Antwerp University, University Hospital, Edegem, Belgium

M.-J. Tassignon et al. (eds.), *Innovative Implantation Technique*,
https://doi.org/10.1007/978-3-030-03086-5_20

3. Clinically insignificant decentration, defined as non-coincident centration of optic and pupil area, though without causing subjective symptoms. Its incidence is estimated to occur in 25% of lens-in-the-bag implantations [2].

Time of onset of IOL malpositioning in the anterior chamber is another parameter that may be used to classify malpositioned IOLs. Initial presentation may range from the time of implantation to a decade or more after the primary surgery. The majority of malpositioned IOLs, however, are observed within 3 months after original surgery [3].

Implant malpositioning may cause significant visual disability mainly due to high-order aberrations, causing decreased contrast sensitivity, glare, monocular diplopia and chromatic distortion. Subjective symptoms associated with a decentred IOL are in correlation with the "aphakic portion" of the pupil. Light passing through this aphakic crescent forms a blurred secondary image on the retina. For example, when 50% of the pupil is exposed, it causes a 50% decrease in contrast [4]. It is important to stress that although most optics are 5.5–6.0 mm in diameter, the effective zone of best acuity may be even smaller, according to the lens design, the lens power and the lens biomaterial (refractive index).

Multifocal implants typically employ a limited central zone for best distance acuity. These IOLs are very sensitive to reduced contrast sensitivity and decreased quality of vision in case of slight IOL decentration. In case of clinically significant lens decentration, patients' subjective complaints include colour discrepancies, observation of the lens haptic/optic and the ability to describe its shape. One paper also described how a patient could observe the pits in the IOL optic after Nd:YAG laser capsulotomy [5, 6].

Over time, the types of malpositioned IOLs have evolved with changes in implant style and surgical technique. Subluxation was most commonly seen with the iris-fixated lenses of the 1970s and 1980s. Pupillary capture of the optic was most common in sulcus-fixated lenses without haptic angulation. Haptic malposition from the posterior chamber into the anterior chamber was often observed through large peripheral iridectomies, still in vogue in the late twentieth century. Elaborate discussions in the literature on sunrise, sunset, and windshield wiper syndromes gave clues about the possible aetiology of this condition. This led to better lens design as well as to improvements in surgical techniques [7]. It is well accepted nowadays that these conditions are associated with the discontinuity of the anterior capsulorhexis, capsular bag tear or loose zonular apparatus, all of which most frequently occur as a complication of cataract surgery [8–10].

However, preexisting conditions that predispose an eye to a weakness of these structures or conditions that restrict the surgeon's view during implantation may lead to a greater likelihood of postoperative IOL malpositioning. Pseudoexfoliation syndrome, prior trauma, prior surgery such as pars plana vitrectomy, systemic connective tissue disease like Marfan's syndrome, extreme advanced age and prior miotic therapy may all increase this risk. This is not to mention the traumatic postoperative dislocation of the IOL, with all of its variable expressions.

20.3 The BIL Implant

The most frequent complication after cataract surgery remains posterior capsule opacification (PCO). The idea of capturing the remaining lens epithelial cells (LECs) in a closed space was based on the laboratory results of Marcantonio and Vrensen [11]. The bag-in-the-lens intraocular lens (BIL-IOL) was designed to eradicate PCO. To achieve this goal, the implantation technique includes an anterior and posterior capsulorhexis of the same size. The insertion of the remaining posterior and anterior capsule into the lens groove of the IOL captures the peripheral LECs, thereby preventing them from migrating onto the visual axis.

The early studies of the bag-in-the-lens implantation showed an incidence of iris capture of 2.35% [12]. Pupil dilation resolved the iris capture in most cases. In the event that it did not, iris capture was resolved at the slit lamp by pushing back the IOL after puncturing the anterior chamber with a 27-gauge needle. In the refractive cases, the iris capture was released in the operating room under topical anaesthesia in association with a peripheral iridotomy. Visual acuity outcome was not affected after the resolution of this complication. Since then, the peripheral groove of the BIL had been reduced to 0.25 mm instead of 0.4 mm, and the haptic flanges were reduced to 0.2 from the initial 0.25 mm, in order to avoid postoperative IOL wobbling.

In unexperienced hands, BIL-IOL dislocation can occur in 0.12% of cases [12]. This complication was a more significant risk prior to the development of the ring caliper in 2007.

Performing a well-sized and centred anterior capsulorhexis was a real challenge before the introduction of different devices that allow for the perfect sizing of the anterior capsulorhexis. The ring caliper, manufactured by Morcher, is the most elegant and subtle tool to help the surgeon to perform a reliable anterior capsulorhexis of the correct size. In addition, it is the less expensive device that is currently on the market for this purpose.

We encountered some cases of lens dislocation after having performed too small anterior and posterior capsulorhexes. Positioning of the BIL in case of too small rhexes demands more pressure and manipulation, increasing the risk to push the lens into the vitreous cavity. One positive is that in the case of BIL diving, it can be repaired by simple vitrectomy. In case of dislocation of the BIL in the presence of too large a rhexis, repositioning is possible provided bean-shaped rings are used to sandwich the BIL. This technique is elaborated more in greater length in other chapters of this book (Nils-Erik Boonstra and Sorcha Ní Dhubhghaill).

In the BIL-IOL technique, the design of the IOL and the sealing of the anterior and posterior capsule, at their merging point, confer a very strong adhesion. In case of trauma, the capsule can release the BIL into the anterior chamber (Fig. 20.1) or into the posterior chamber (Fig. 20.2), leaving the capsular bag intact. The seal around the lens makes it act like a release valve for the traumatic shockwave and generally leaves the zonulae undisturbed. This allows a unique opportunity and advantage to reposition the BIL very easily in its original location. The BIL can be

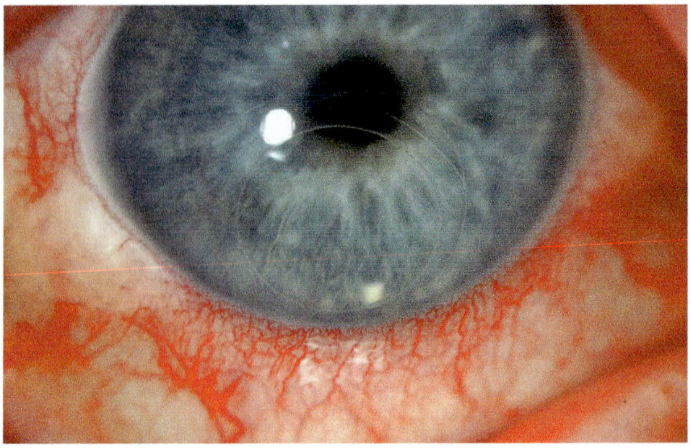

Fig. 20.1 Anterior luxation of the BIL after blunt ocular trauma

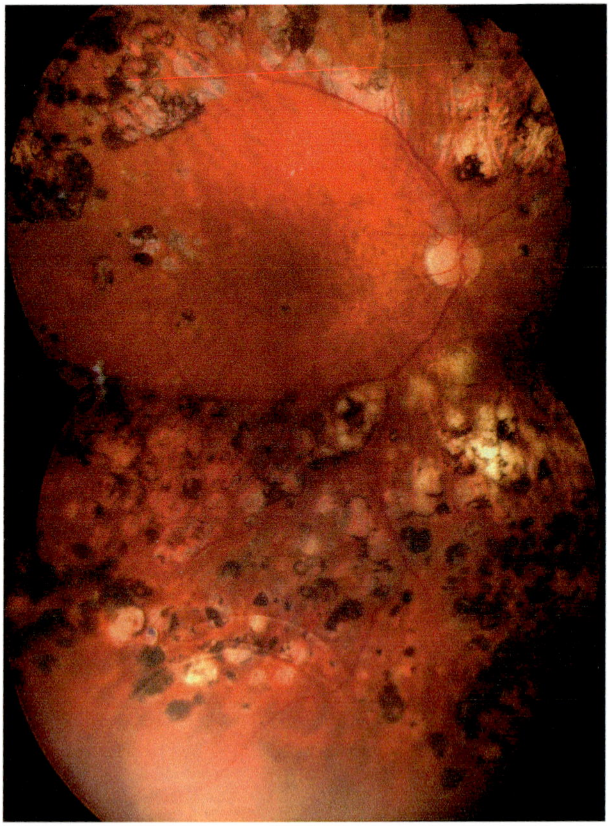

Fig. 20.2 Dropped BIL in the posterior segment of the eye in a vitrectomized eye before the advent of the ring caliper

repositioned into its original position under local anaesthesia. This technique gives by far less complications than putting a traditional posterior chamber IOL into the anterior chamber [13]. In cases of combined BIL and vitrectomy with gas insufflation, we tend to use the 89F model that has a larger anterior plate. This reduces the risk for iris incarceration and posterior dislocation (this technique is elaborated in greater length in the chapter by Tillman Eckert).

References

1. Panton R, Sulewski M, Parker J, Panton P, Stark W. Surgical management of subluxed posterior-chamber intraocular lenses. Arch Ophthalmol. 1993;111(7):919–26.
2. Smiddy W, Ibanez G, Alfonso E, Flynn H Jr. Surgical management of dislocated intraocular lenses. J Cataract Refract Surg. 1995;21(1):64–9.
3. Shakin E, Carty J Jr. Clinical management of posterior chamber intraocular lens implants dislocated in the vitreous cavity. Ophthalmic Surg Lasers. 1995;26(6):529–34.
4. Kumar S, Miller D. Effect of intraocular decentration on retinal image contrast. J Cataract Refract Surg. 1990;16(6):712–4.
5. Miedziak A, Carty J Jr. Chromatic visual phenomenon caused by a subluxed intraocular lens. J Cataract Refract Surg. 1996;22(5):637–8.
6. Yong V, Lee H, AuEong K, Yong V. Subjective visual perception of a dislocated intraocular lens. J Cataract Refract Surg. 2002;28(8):1494–5.
7. Smith S, Lindstrom R. Malpositioned posterior chamber lenses: etiology, prevention, and management. J Am Intraocular Implant Soc. 1985;11:584–91.
8. Petersen A, Bluth L, Campion M. Delayed posterior dislocation of silicone plate-haptic lenses after neodymium: YAG capsulotomy. J Cataract Refract Surg. 2000;26(12):1827–9.
9. Agustin A, Miller K. Posterior dislocation of a plate-haptic silicone intraocular lens with large fixation holes. J Cataract Refract Surg. 2000;26(9):1428–9.
10. Schneiderman T, Johnson M, Smiddy W, Flynn H Jr, Bennet S, Cantrill H. Surgical management of posteriorly dislocated silicone plate haptic intraocular lenses. Am J Ophthalmol. 1997;123(5):629–35.
11. Marcantonio JM, Vrensen GFJM. Cell biology of posterior capsular opacification. Eye. 1999;13:484–8.
12. Tassignon MJ, Gobin L, Mathysen D, Van Looveren J, De Groot V. Clinical outcomes of cataract surgery after bag-in-the-lens intraocular lens implantation following ISO standard 11979-7: 2006. J Cataract Refract Surg. 2011;37(12):2120–9.
13. Liu J, Koch D, Emery J. Complications of implanting three-piece C-loop posterior chamber lenses in the anterior chamber. Ophthalmic Surg. 1988;19(11):802–7.

Preparing Pediatric Cataract Patients for BIL Cataract Surgery

21

L. Lytvynchuk, D. Kuhn, M. Sander, and B. Lorenz

21.1 Introduction

Pediatric lens disorders, despite being by and large treatable, remain one of the major causes of visual disability in children. When left untreated, they usually lead to the development of amblyopia or even blindness [1, 2]. In high-income countries, pediatric cataracts have become one of the most commonly avoidable causes of blindness in children [2]. The impact of visual impairment on children and on their quality of life, both socially and economically, is considered to be tremendous [3]. Each year nearly 0.5 million children develop blindness, which is caused by different ocular and systemic diseases including lens disorders [4, 5]. It has been reported that over 200,000 children worldwide are blind from cataracts and that this rate is increasing among the already 1.4 million blind children in the world [4]. Global vision's 2020 initiative included childhood blindness among priority eye diseases and established the Global Childhood Blindness Program [6]. That is why the adequate and time-conscious management of pediatric lens disorders is essential.

There are two major groups of pediatric lens disorders: pediatric cataract and dislocation of the crystalline lens. Both entities usually require a complex treatment approach, including proper and early diagnosis, therapeutic treatment or surgical intervention, and visual and social rehabilitation. In this chapter, we will focus on the necessary preoperative considerations regarding pediatric cataract surgery.

L. Lytvynchuk · B. Lorenz (✉)
Department of Ophthalmology, Justus-Liebig-University and Universitaetsklinikum Giessen and Marburg GmbH, Campus Giessen, Giessen, Germany
e-mail: lyubomyr.lytvynchuk@augen.med.uni-giessen.de; birgit.lorenz@uniklinikum-giessen.de

D. Kuhn · M. Sander
Department of Anaesthesiology, Justus-Liebig-University and Universitaetsklinikum Giessen and Marburg GmbH, Campus Giessen, Giessen, Germany
e-mail: detlef.F.Kuhn@chiru.med.uni-giessen.de; Michael.Sander@chiru.med.uni-giessen.de

M.-J. Tassignon et al. (eds.), *Innovative Implantation Technique*,
https://doi.org/10.1007/978-3-030-03086-5_21

21.2 Epidemiology

The epidemiology of pediatric cataracts depends on various factors that should be assessed in each particular population group. The thorough analysis of the causes and overview of the rate of the pathology is important for establishing preventive methods and the best and most optimal approaches in treatment. The most important factors that influence the epidemiology of pediatric cataract include economic development, the population's cultural specifics, dietary conditions, and level of pediatric medical care [6, 7]. Prenatal rubella infection remains an important cause of pediatric cataract in many developing countries all over the world [6]. The prevalence of pediatric cataracts is increasing in some countries, as a result of the earlier detection of cataracts because of improved screening through the Vision 2020 program [8].

21.3 Etiology

The etiology of pediatric cataract is determined by multiple pathophysiological factors [9–11]. It can be classified into hereditary, non-hereditary, and idiopathic types. The frequency of all three cataract types varies in different countries and population groups [9]. The results of a Danish Study published in 2004, which included 1027 cases, showed that the most frequent type was an idiopathic form of cataract involved in 63% of cases [12]. The frequency of hereditary and non-hereditary pediatric cataracts in this study was calculated as 29% and 8% of cases, respectively. Hereditary cataracts are related to gene mutations or familial inheritance. The most common mutations are observed in crystalline genes, membrane protein genes, and cytoskeletal protein genes [9, 13]. This type of cataract can also be related to faulty developmental regulation or other ocular or systemic abnormalities [14]. The non-hereditary pediatric cataracts are usually associated with various etiologies, such as metabolic disorders (diabetes, galactosemia, hypoglycemia, and galactokinase deficiency), intrauterine infection (TORCH), ocular trauma, and radiation or iatrogenic causes [15, 16].

The diagnosis of idiopathic cataract can be established when the exact cause of the lens disorder cannot be detected. It is estimated that the majority of unilateral cataract cases, and nearly half of all bilateral cataract cases, have an idiopathic origin [7]. Additionally, pediatric cataracts can be defined by the age of onset as congenital (within 1 year of life) or juvenile cataract (within the first decade) [9]. Moreover, congenital cataract may be associated with one of the systemic syndromes that affect the musculoskeletal system (Smith–Lemli–Opitz and Stickler, myotonic dystrophy) [17, 18], central nervous system (Marinesco–Sjögren, Zellweger), kidney (Lowe syndrome, Alport syndrome, and Hallerman–Streiff–François syndrome) [19–21], or skin (Cockayne, incontinentia pigmenti, ichthyosis) [22]. It has been reported by different authors that in between 8.3% and 25% of congenital cataracts have an inherited origin [23].

21.4 Timing of Surgery

Visual outcomes following cataract surgery in children are strongly correlated with the period of visual deprivation caused by the opaque crystalline lens [24, 25]. Visual deprivation and its duration need to be considered in relation to the period of visual development during which the deprivation began. The concept of latent, plastic, and critical periods was introduced in order to define the age at which the development of the visual system is most vulnerable. Based on laboratory and clinical studies, it was established that the critical period can last from birth to 12 years [26]. It is also believed that there are different sensitive periods for each visual function [27]. Generally, the sensitive period of visual development remains most plastic until 2–3 years, with a gradual decrease of plasticity up until 9–12 years. Throughout the latent period, the visual deprivation causes little or no effect on visual potential. During the sensitive period, with decreased plasticity, the visual deprivation usually causes permanent and irreversible changes in the development of the affected eye's visual function. It has been shown that in cases of congenital cataract, when the deprivation persists from birth, the latent period ends after 6 weeks of age [28–30]. In order to avoid significant anomalies of visual development, performing cataract surgery within 6 weeks is recommended. The same timing of surgery is employed for cases of unilateral congenital cataract [29, 31]. Hartmann et al. have reported on the results of a randomized multicenter clinical trial for 114 infants (Infant Aphakia Treatment Study Group) based on the examinations performed at the age of 4.5 years with primary surgery aged between 1 and 7 months. The authors concluded that early surgery is important to obtaining good visual outcomes in pediatric patients with unilateral infantile cataracts [32]. For bilateral cases, the optimal age for cataract removal is 8 weeks, given that surgery is performed after 10 weeks of age and results in a visual acuity of ≤20/100 [33]. Studies have shown a bilinear correlation of visual outcome and age at surgery in patients with bilateral congenital cataract, which was characterized by a progressive decrease in visual acuity with increasing age [34]. Additionally, attention has to be paid to the risks of local and general complications by pediatric patients of different ages [35].

It is reasonable to schedule the surgery at the earliest time of deprivation and, at the same time, within the plastic period of visual development, when the distorted visual functions still can be fully or partially repaired [9]. However, there is a higher risk of postoperative complications when the surgery is performed at a younger age [36]. Overall, the decision regarding the timing of the surgery has to be based on the clinical condition and the presence of significant visual deprivation.

21.5 Indications for Surgery

The indications for the surgery can differ in every particular case, but surgery is usually suggested in the following cases: complete lens opacifications, central opacifications (≥3 mm in diameter) that occlude the visual axis, and substantial visual deprivation associated with nystagmus or strabismus [37]. The development of the visual functions in children is strongly correlated with the clarity of optical media. That is why early surgical intervention has to be considered. Conversely, a newborn's eyes that have congenital cataracts are underdeveloped, and the ocular response to the surgery can lead to the development of postoperative complications. Determining the timing of the surgery, by taking all of the patient's existing peculiarities into account, is recommended.

21.6 IOL Selection

At present, the surgical treatment of pediatric cataracts with the implantation of an IOL is a widely accepted approach [7, 9, 11, 35]. However, IOL selection and power calculation in children are more challenging compared to adults. The fact that the anatomical parameters of the child's eye are constantly changing (axial length, corneal curvature and diameter, ciliary body, capsular bag) makes the prediction of postoperative refraction in different ages a very difficult task. Additionally, inaccuracies of biometrical parameters usually achieved in the operating room (misalignment of the eye, deformation of the soft cornea, handheld diagnostic tools, etc.) can lead to errors in the IOL power calculations, which will definitely affect postoperative refraction. The choice of IOL power usually depends on the surgeon's tactics with regard to target refraction and methods to treat postoperative amblyopia. The standard formulas for IOL power calculation in adults have been used for children as well. The most frequently used formulas are those that require AL and corneal power (SRK-T, Hoffer Q, Haigis, Holladay). It has been shown by multiple studies that the prediction error after IOL implantation in children is higher than in adults by using the same formulas for IOL power calculation, ranging from 1.22 D to 1.64 D [38–40]. The role of IOL implantation in the treatment of postoperative amblyopia is not clear. However, the studies that showed no significant difference in visual functions between aphakic and pseudophakic eyes have analyzed the lens-in-the-bag technique or primary implantation of the IOL in the sulcus [32, 41]. Moreover, a complex of anisometropic changes (aniseikonia, anisophoria, anisometropia, age fluctuations, amblyopia treatment) have to be considered in cases of unilateral cataracts [10]. It has been shown that the myopic shift (myopisation) is larger after the implantation of an IOL with higher power comparing to a lowly powered IOL. At present, there are no clear data about the best strategy for postoperative target refraction in long-term follow-up; however, there are a number of recommendation tables regarding postoperative refraction.

21.7 Surgical Approach

Various surgical techniques are available that use different types of IOL to treat cataracts in children. The most common approach is to perform a posterior capsulorhexis in order to avoid the risk of posterior capsule reopacification (PCO). Additionally, the optic capture technique is used in order to prevent retrolental reopacification [42]. It has been claimed that a sharp-edged lens-in-the-bag IOL prevents the migration of the lens epithelial cells, but the occurrence of PCO in long-term follow-up has also been reported [43]. PCO has been reported in up to 80% of eyes that have cataract extraction with IOL implantation, depending on the length of the follow-up [43, 44]. The bag-in-the-lens technique, first reported by Tassignon et al., has revolutionized the surgical approach and has decreased the rate of major postoperative complications [45]. The most important advantages of the BIL IOLs are that this technique facilitates the optimal centration of the optical part of the IOL and that correct implantation drastically minimizes the rate of visual axis reopacification (VAR). This is achieved through the special IOL design, where the rims of the posterior and anterior capsulorhexis are captured inside the groove of the BIL IOL, thereby limiting the escape trajectory for posterior lens opacities [45].

21.8 Preoperative Assessment

The assessment of the visual functions in preoperative and postoperative periods in children remains challenging. There are a number of parameters that have to be studied. Apart from visual acuity, examining fixation, nystagmus (frequency, amplitude, direction of the beat, waveform), eye alignment, and color vision has all been suggested. Furthermore, it is important to realize that visual function is not solely dependent on the ophthalmic status.

Almost every cataract surgery in children necessitates general anesthesia [46] (Fig. 21.1). With the development of modern surgical techniques, cataract surgery in children has become a relatively safe and quick technique. Congenital cataracts may be associated with various systemic syndromes, which can make it difficult to give a prognosis on the results of anesthesia. The impact of general anesthesia on neuro-ophthalmological pathways has not been profoundly studied, in spite of the fact that this could play a role in the postoperative visual outcomes.

21.9 The Role of General Anesthesia

There has been a growing debate on the topic of avoiding repeated general anesthesia for elective surgery in children under the age of 2 years in recent years because of a possible link between anesthetics and neurobehavioral effects [47–49], which led to an FDA safety announcement in 2016 [50]. Remarkably safe general anesthesia is administered to millions of pediatric patients worldwide every year. Since there is not enough information about the effects of anesthetic drugs on the brains of infants, nobody really knows whether the use of these medicines poses a risk or if the risk is significant enough to outweigh the benefits of the planned surgery. It is unlikely that the surgery itself has a detrimental effect on the neurobehavioral outcome of children operated upon, given that pediatric lens surgery is considered "minimally invasive surgery" with very little surgical trauma. This is especially true if the ophthalmic surgery is of a short duration. Anesthetics are a necessary part of

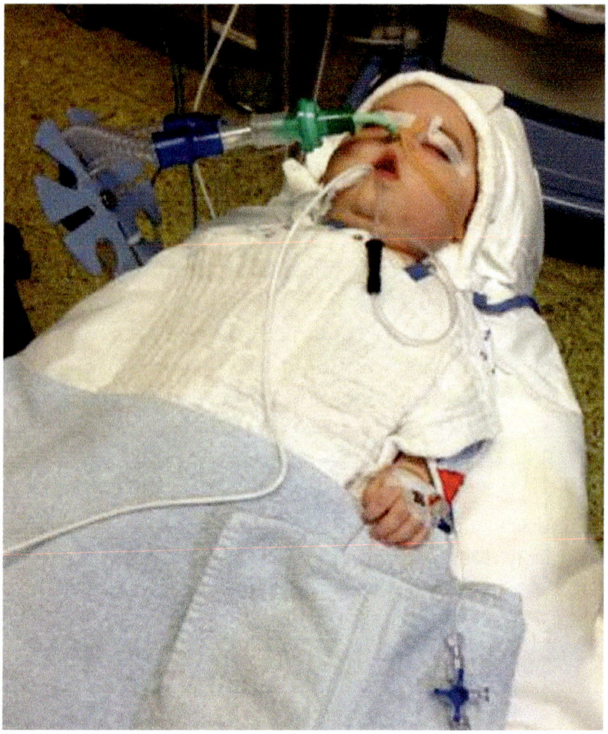

Fig. 21.1 Positioning of the pediatric patient

the care of children needing any surgery or procedures. It should be noted that in animal studies almost all anesthetics have been found to cause injuries to the brain at some point. Therefore, specific medications or techniques can hardly be considered to be any safer or better than any others [51, 52].

For some children who have been scheduled for lens surgery, the ophthalmic problem is merely just one aspect of a systemic disease complex. The parents are usually best informed about the medical history of their children and can contribute thoroughly both to the preoperative evaluation and to the physical examination [53].

As mentioned previously, congenital cataract can be associated with a variety of systemic hereditary diseases, such as homocystinuria, Marfan syndrome, Down syndrome, etc. Despite cataract surgery being a "minimally invasive procedure," the anamnesis has to include a full medical and surgical history [54]. Pneumonia, laryngitis, and acute asthma are clear indications that surgery should be delayed by at least 4 weeks [55, 56].

General anesthesia presents severe risks in a very small number of children with severe comorbidity. Explaining the whole anesthetic procedure to the parents is mandatory, and this should include possible side effects and complications related to the anesthesia. Far more importantly, from the point of view of the children at least, are their concerns about pain induced by venipuncture, postoperative pain, and the discomfort caused by an eye patch (Fig. 21.2). All of those aspects should be addressed before asking for consent.

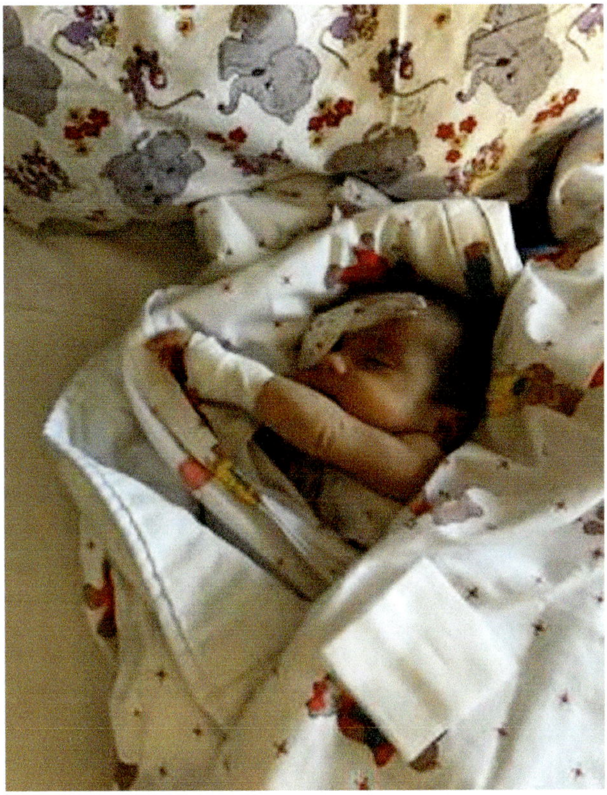

Fig. 21.2 Postoperative eye shield

21.10 Conclusion

In recent years, ophthalmic surgeons have widened the indication for planned lens surgery in infants under the age of 3 years. It is important to consider all factors related to the cataract thoroughly: the patient's age, presence of other ocular or systemic pathology, the different aspects of visual function, etc. It is unlikely that the surgery itself has a detrimental effect on the neurobehavioral outcome of operated children, given that pediatric lens surgery is considered a "minimally invasive surgery" with very little surgical trauma. Unfortunately, this may not be true of the general anesthesia needed to perform this kind of surgery in neonates or infants. Based on review results in 2016, the FDA released a safety announcement warning that repeated use of general anesthetic and sedation drugs during surgeries in children younger than 3 years may affect the development of children's brains. Healthcare professionals, and anesthesiologists in particular, have to discuss those warnings with parents, thereby carefully balancing the benefits of appropriate anesthesia in young children against the potential risks. A comprehensive medical history, a laboratory, and an extended examination are important in young patients that suffer from complex syndromes.

21.11 Core Messages

- Adequate development of visual functions and optimal visual outcomes are the main goals of pediatric cataract surgery.
- The advantages of both, aphakia and pseudophakia, remain debatable.
- The impact of general anesthesia on neurobehavioral issues and visual outcomes is not well studied, so care should be taken to limit general anesthesia to the minimum needed.
- The bag-in-the-lens technique allows for the minimization of the rate of visual axis reopacification after cataract surgery.
- The preferable method of IOL calculation and the long-term visual outcomes have to be studied further.

References

1. Solebo AL, Teoh L, Rahi J. Epidemiology of blindness in children. Arch Dis Child. 2017. pii: archdischild-2016-310532.
2. Lenhart PD, Courtright P, Wilson ME, et al. Global challenges in the management of congenital cataract: proceedings of the 4th international congenital cataract symposium held on March 7, 2014, New York, New York. J AAPOS. 2015;19:e1–e8. 47.
3. Vinluan ML, Olveda RM, Olveda DU, et al. Access to essential paediatric eye surgery in the developing world: a case of congenital cataracts left untreated. BMJ Case Rep. 2015;2015:bcr2014208197. 45.
4. Foster A, Gilbert C. Epidemiology of childhood blindness. Eye. 1992;6:173–6.
5. Wilson ME, Pandey SK, Thakur J. Paediatric cataract blindness in the developing world: surgical techniques and intraocular lenses in the new millennium. Br J Ophthalmol. 2003;87(1):14–9.
6. World Health Organisation. Global initiative for the elimination of avoidable blindness. WHO, Geneva, publication no.PBL/ 97.61. 1977.
7. Chan WH, Biswas S, Ashworth JL, Lloyd C. Congenital and infantile cataract: aetiology and management. Eur J Pediatr. 2012;171:625–30.
8. Lin D, Chen J, Lin Z, et al. 10-Year overview of the hospital-based prevalence and treatment of congenital cataracts: the CCPMOH experience. PLoS One. 2015;10:e0142298. 46.
9. Liu Y. Pediatric Lens diseases. Singapore: Springer; 2017. p. 29–54.
10. Wilson M, Trivedi R. Pediatric cataract surgery: techniques, complications and management. Philadelphia: Wolters Kluwer; 2014.
11. Nucci P. Pediatric Cataract. Basel: Karger; 2016.
12. Haargaard B, Wohlfahrt J, Fledelius HC, Rosenberg T, Melbye M, editors. A nationwide Danish study of 1027 cases of congenital/infantile cataracts: etiological and clinical classifications. Ophthalmology. 2004;111(12):2292–8.
13. Francois J. Genetics of cataract. Ophthalmologica. 1982;184:61–71. [PubMed: 7063172] 15.
14. Kuhli-Hattenbach C, Hofmann C, Wenner Y, Koch F, Kohnen T. Congenital cataract surgery without intraocular lens implantation in persistent fetal vasculature syndrome: long-term clinical and functional results. J Cataract Refract Surg. 2016;42:759–67.
15. Stambolian D. Galactose and cataract. Surv Ophthalmol. 1988;32:33–49.
16. Stambolian D, Ai Y, Sikjanin D, Nesburn K, Sathe G, Rosenberg M, Bergsma DJ. Cloning of the galactokinase cDNA and identification of two families with galacktokinase deficiency and cataracts. Nat Genet. 1995;10:307–12.
17. Cotlier E, Rice P. Cataracts in the Smith–Lemli–Opitz syndrome. Am J Ophthalmol. 1971;72:955–9.

18. Fold DH, Weingiest TA, editors. The eye in systemic disease. Philadelphia: JB Lippincott; 1990.
19. Falls HF, Schull WJ. Hallerman–Streiff syndrome. A dyscephaly with congenital cataracts and hypotrichsis. Arch Ophthalmol. 1960;63:409–20.
20. Jacobs M, Jeffret B, Kriss A, Taylor D, Sa G, Barrat M. Ophthalmologic assessment of young patients with Alport syndrome. Ophthalmology. 1992;99:1039–44.
21. Tripathi RC, Cibis GW, Tripathi BJ. Pathogenesis of cataracts in patients with Lowes syndrome. Ophthalmology. 1986;93:1046–51.
22. Pearce WG. Ocular and genetic features of Cockaynes syndrome. Can J Ophthalmol. 1972;7:435–44.
23. Merin S. Inherited cataracts. In: Merin S, editor. Inherited eye diseases. New York: Marcel Dekker,Inc; 1991. p. 86–120.
24. Moreira J, Ribeiro I, Mota Á, Gonçalves R, Coelho P, Maio T, Tenedório P. Pediatric cataracts: a retrospective study of 12 years (2004–2016). Acta Med Port. 2017;30(3):169–74.
25. Eriksen JR, Bronsard A, Mosha M, et al. Predictors of poor follow-up in children that had cataract surgery. Ophthalmic Epidemiol. 2006;13:237–43.
26. Hubel DH, Wiesel TN. The period of susceptibility to the physiological effects of unilateral eye closure in kittens. J Physiol. 1970;206(2):419436.
27. Lewis TL, Maurer D. Multiple sensitive periods in human visual development: evidence from visual deprived children. Dev Psychobiol. 2005;46(3):163–83.
28. Birch EE, Cheng C, Stager DR Jr, Weakley DR Jr, Stager DR. The critical period for surgical treatment of dense congenital bilateral cataracts. J AAPOS. 2009;13(1):67–71.
29. Birch EE, Stager DR. The critical period for surgical treatment of dense congenital unilateral cataract. Invest Ophthalmol Vis Sci. 1996;37:1532–8.
30. Birch EE, Cheng C, Stager DR, Felius J. Visual acuity development after the implantation of unilateral intraocular lenses in infants and young children. J AAPOS. 2005;9:527–32.
31. Bradford G, Keech RV, Scott W. Factors affecting visual outcome after surgery for bilateral congenital cataracts. Am J Ophthalmol. 1994;117:58–64.
32. Eugenie Hartmann E, Lynn MJ, Lambert SR, for the Infant Aphakia Treatment Study Group. Baseline characteristics of the infant Aphakia treatment study population: predicting recognition acuity at 4.5 years of age. Invest Ophthalmol Vis Sci. 2015;56:388–95.
33. Lambert SR, Lynn MJ, Reeves R, Plager DA, Buckley EG, Wilson ME. Is there a latent period for the surgical treatment of children with dense bilateral congenital cataracts? J AAPOS. 2006;10(1):3036.
34. Birch EE, Cheng C, Stager DR Jr, Weakley DR Jr, Stager DR Sr. The critical period for surgical treatment of dense congenital bilateral cataracts. J AAPOS. 2008;13:6771.
35. M. Edward Wilson, MD Pediatric Cataracts: Overview https://www.aao.org/pediatric-center-detail/pediatric-cataracts-overview. Nov 11 2015.
36. Kuhli-Hattenbach C, Fronius M, Kohnen T. Impact of timing of surgery on outcome in children with bilateral congenital cataract. Ophthalmologe. 2017;114(3):252–8. https://doi.org/10.1007/s00347-016-0326-5.
37. Zetterstrom C, Lundvall A, Kugelberg M. Cataracts in children. J Cataract Refract Surg. 2005;31:824–40.
38. Mezer E, Rootman DS, Abdolell M, Levin AV. Early postoperative refractive outcomes of pediatric intraocular lens implantation. J Cataract Refract Surg. 2004;30(3):603–10.
39. Andreo LK, Wilson ME, Saunders RA. Predictive value of regression and theoretical IOL formulas in pediatric intraocular lens implantation. J Pediatr Ophthalmol Strabismus. 1997;34(4):240–3.
40. Moore DB, Ben Zion I, Neely DE, Roberts GJ, Sprunger DT, Plager DA. Refractive outcomes with secondary intraocular lens implantation in children. J AAPOS. 2009;13(6):551–4.
41. McClatchey SK, Dahan E, Maselli E, Gimbel HV, Wilson ME, Lambert SR, Buckley EG, Freedman SF, Plager DA, Parks MM. A comparison of the rate of refractive growth in pediatric aphakic and pseudophakic eyes. Ophthalmology. 2000;107(1):118–22.

42. Gimbel HV. Posterior capsulorhexis with optic capture in pediatric cataract and intraocular lens surgery. Ophthalmology. 1996;103(11):1871–5.
43. Apple DJ, Solomon KD, Tetz MR, et al. Posterior capsule opacification. Surv Ophthalmol. 1992;37:73–116.
44. Ohadi C, Moreira H, McDonnell P. Posterior capsule opacification. Curr Opin Ophthalmol. 1991;2:46–52.
45. Tassignon MJ, De Groot V, Vrensen GF. Bag-in-the-lens implantation of intraocular lenses. J Cataract Refract Surg. 2002;28:1182–8.
46. Gayer S, Tutiven J. Anesthesia for pediatric ocular surgery. Ophthalmol Clin North Am. 2006;19(2):269–78.
47. Andropoulos DB, Greene MF. Anesthesia and developing brains — implications of the FDA warning. N Engl J Med. 2017;376:905–7.
48. Loepke AW, Soriano SG. An assessment of the effects of general anesthetics on developing brain structure and neurocognitive function. Anesth Analg. 2008;106:1681–707.
49. Korkman M, Kemp SL, Kirk U. Effects of age on neurocognitive measures of children ages 5 to 12: a cross-sectional study on 800 children from the United States. Dev Neuropsychol. 2001;20:331–54.
50. U.S. Food and Drug Administration (FDA), Safety Announcement. FDA review results in new warnings about using general anesthetics and sedation drugs in young children and pregnant women. [12-14-2016].
51. Briner A, De Roo M, Dayer A, Muller D, Habre W, Vutskits L. Volatile anesthetics rapidly increase dendritic spine density in the rat medial prefrontal cortex during synaptogenesis. Anesthesiology. 2010;112:546–56.
52. Creeley C, Dikranian K, Dissen G, Martin L, Olney J, Brambrink A. Propofol- induced apoptosis of neurones and oligodendrocytes in fetal and neonatal rhesus macaque brain. Br J Anaesth. 2013;110(Suppl 1):i29–38.
53. Morrison A. Ophthalmology, plastics, oncology, radiology, thoracic, and dental surgery. In: Doyle E, editor. Paediatric anaesthesia. Oxford: Oxford University Press; 2007. p. 298–307.
54. Crick RP, Khaw PT. A textbook of clinical ophthalmology, A practical guide to disorders of the eyes and their managements. 2nd ed. Copyright 1997 By World Scientific Publishing Co. Pte. Ltd.
55. Van der Walt J. Anesthesia in children with viral respiratory tract infections. Paediatr Anaesth. 1995;5:257–61.
56. Shemesh S, Tamir S, Goldfarb A, Ezri T, Roth Y. To proceed or not to proceed: ENT surgery in paediatric patients with acute upper respiratory tract infection. J Laryngol Otol. 2016;130(9):800–4.

Visual Outcomes and Complications After BIL in the Paediatric Population

22

L. Lytvynchuk and B. Lorenz

22.1 Visual Outcomes

Testing and interpreting children's visual function remains challenging. The results of various visual tests depend, first and foremost, on the patient's age and attention, time of examination, examiner's experience, etc. [1]. The postoperative visual outcomes after cataract surgery in children depend on the age of onset, associated ocular and/or systemic pathology, timing of the surgery, surgical technique and target refraction; these can all be influenced by a variety of systemic and local complications. Independently, the efficacy of postoperative visual rehabilitation will be greatly influential on the long-term results.

Postoperative visual outcomes are greatly determined by the target refraction of the eye treated and the power of the IOL implanted. However, it is not clear yet how to achieve this in an exact way in a paediatric population. Axial length (AL) and keratometry measurements are usually performed under general anaesthesia using handheld devices in infants and toddlers or in disabled children. Different formulas for the calculation of IOL power are currently used, even though the accuracy of IOL power calculation in children younger than 36 months remains questionable [2, 3].

The most common complications that affect visual function include posterior capsule opacities (PCO), secondary glaucoma, loss of anterior vitreous and cystoid macular oedema [4]. PCO, with excessive retrolental cellular proliferation, remains the main concern for the postoperative clarity of the visual axis and for visual recovery. Intraoperative capsulorhexis has become a standard step in paediatric cataract surgery, one that significantly reduces the rate of PCO. However, a partial or complete

L. Lytvynchuk · B. Lorenz (✉)
Department of Ophthalmology, Justus-Liebig-University, Giessen and Universitaetsklinikum Giessen and Marburg GmbH, Campus Giessen, Giessen, Germany
e-mail: lyubomyr.lytvynchuk@augen.med.uni-giessen.de; birgit.lorenz@uniklinikum-giessen.de

M.-J. Tassignon et al. (eds.), *Innovative Implantation Technique*,
https://doi.org/10.1007/978-3-030-03086-5_22

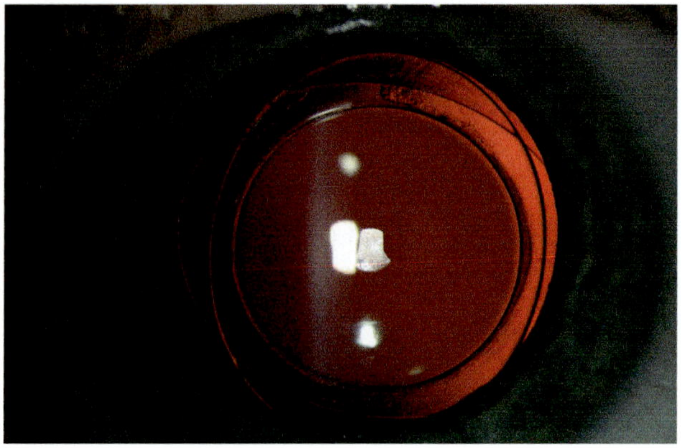

Fig. 22.1 Postoperative image of a BIL IOL implanted at age 7 years

closure of the posterior capsule occurs in up to 40% of cases, thereby leading to a decrease of visual axis clarity, as well as to decreased visual function [5–9].

The use of the bag-in-the-lens technique in paediatric cataract cases allows for the visual axis to remain free of secondary opacification and for the optimal optic condition for the development of visual functions (Fig. 22.1). The correct placement of the BIL IOL facilitates good centration and the stability of the IOL in the posterior chamber, both of which are major factors in the achievement of optimal refractive results. The BIL IOL implantation technique was first performed in adults and has demonstrated both a high success rate and a low frequency of postoperative posterior capsular opacities (PCO) [10, 11].

The bag-in-the-lens technique necessitates a learning curve, with little or no additional consumption of time if performed by an experienced surgeon. An additional transcorneal or pars plana vitrectomy can sometimes be needed in paediatric cataract cases. This can be necessary due to the prolapse of the vitreous body, presence of persistent fetal vasculature (PFV) or abnormalities of the anterior vitreolenticular interface.

Currently, there are limited data available regarding postoperative short-term and long-term visual outcomes after cataract surgery in children using the BIL technique, but it is increasingly used throughout the world. The authors believe that the analysis of visual functions has to be performed in single age groups, given that the causes of cataract and progression of postoperative development of visual functions differ.

22.1.1 Postoperative Visual Rehabilitation

The development of the visual system starts in the postnatal period and continues up into one's teenage years. The presence of sufficient external stimuli after birth is critical for future visual acuity and binocular vision, as well as to the adequate growth of visual pathways and the optical system. The treatment of paediatric cataracts can be divided into two stages. The first stage involves the surgical removal of the cataract, with IOL implantation in the case of the BIL technique. The second stage of treatment involves the correction of the remaining refractive error and the treatment of amblyopia.

Correction of Residual Refractive Error All paediatric patients, who have undergone uneventful cataract surgery, have to start postoperative visual rehabilitation, ideally within a few days after the surgery. The normal growth of the eye is characterized by an increase in axial length and decrease of the corneal curvature; the reason why is that refraction will evolve from hypermetropia to emmetropia or even myopia over time. This is why the IOL is calculated to achieve postoperative hypermetropia in infants and toddlers. However, the unfocused light is not enough to provide an optimal stimulus to the retina, which is essential for the visual function's early development. The early postoperative correction of the residual refractive error is, therefore, strongly recommended in infants and toddlers for near distance.

The timing of the surgical intervention in paediatric cataract patients and the start of amblyopia treatment including the correction of the residual refractive error are crucial with regard to the sensitive and critical period of visual development in children. This is especially so in cases of congenital cataract.

Residual refractive errors are corrected with glasses or contact lenses (CL), but both kinds of correction can fail due to insufficient compliance. Correction with glasses is usually prescribed in cases of binocular cataract or in children who cannot tolerate contact lenses. Modern paediatric glasses are relatively safe and the lenses can be replaced easily if damaged. The possibility of bifocal lenses is one of the advantages of glasses. However, there are some disadvantages related to correction with glasses. Stable fixation of the glasses is difficult in patients under 1 year due to the relative weight of the glasses and to difficulties in keeping the frame in place on the child's nose bridge and ears, although very satisfactory frames have become available in recent years. The possible influence of spherical and colour aberrations of the glasses on a child's visual system has to be considered as well, although this has not been well-studied in the paediatric population. Moreover, the difference in magnification, which cannot be predicted precisely, can cause aniseikonia and impact the fusion of the visual inputs, which is crucial for the development and maintenance of binocular vision. The small square of the lenses in the glasses and its frame make the visual fields smaller and impair the focus on the paracentral and peripheral retina.

In contrast, CL eliminate the risk for aniseikonia, due to their firm contact with the cornea and absence of magnification or reduction of visual input size. The use of CL markedly reduces the inconveniences related to the use of glasses, such as the limitation of activity, discomfort to the ears and nose and the risk of damaging with consequent eye injury. Additionally, corneal astigmatism can be corrected more efficiently with the use of CL that have to be of a rigid type in the case of astigmatism. Children cannot usually express the early complaints caused by contact lenses. Therefore, attention has to be paid to possible complications related to CL, such as corneal inflammation, local allergic reactions, corneal trauma due to damaged CL, dry eye and corneal hypoxia. It is recommended to avoid anisometropia, given that an interocular difference in refraction of more than 2.0 D can lead to the development of amblyopia. The power of the CL prescribed depends on the patient's age and the preferred distance to be corrected. In patients under 1 year, the near vision is more important; therefore, an overcorrection ranging from 2.0 D to 3.5 D is recommended. The need for overcorrection decreases with age, and emmetropia is recommended at the age of about 4, together with bifocals or even progressive lenses.

In our practice, children under 1 year are corrected for near vision. Optical correction should be provided for both, near and distance, in children over 2 years old.

Correction with bifocal glasses is strongly recommended in children aged 2–6 years old who have undergone bilateral cataract surgery. The prescription of progressive glasses can be considered in children older than 6 years.

Treatment of Amblyopia In spite of the low rate of intra- and postoperative complications after BIL technique, all paediatric patients remain at risk for the development or persistence of amblyopia, which is the most frequent cause of monocular visual impairment in children with an incidence rate of 2–5%. The importance of amblyopia treatment is supported by data revealing that acquired ocular pathology, such as inflammatory diseases or ocular trauma, is more likely to occur on the fellow eye. After the paediatric cataract has been removed, some possible causes of amblyopia can still remain. Suppression, inadequate motility of the eye, reduced fixation, aniseikonia, anisometropia and strabismus are possible factors leading to the development and exacerbation of amblyopia. Therefore, the treatment of amblyopia has to be started as soon as possible.

Occlusion is one of the most effective approaches to treating amblyopia. It allows one to diminish the dominance of the better eye and for a decrease in suppression of the amblyopic eye. The occlusion regime is prescribed individually and depends on multiple factors, such as age, presence of strabismus, pre- and postoperative vision in both the dominant and the non-dominant eye or the degree of suppression. Occlusion of the leading eye in patients up to 1 year of age can be necessary during half of their waking time.

Moreover, strabismus surgery may be necessary to allow for the development or restoration of binocular vision, which is essential for visual outcomes.

22.1.2 Short-Term Visual Outcomes (0–1 Year)

In 2007, Tassignon et al. first reported the results of a multicentre study on BIL IOL implantation in 32 eyes of 22 paediatric patients with a mean age of 6 years and 2 months (range 2 months to 14 years) [12]. IOL power was calculated prior to the surgery. The mean postoperative follow-up period was 17.45 months (range 4.0–68.8 months). The target refraction was +6.0 D in patients younger than 1 year, +4.0 D between 1 and 2 years, and emmetropia in children over 2. The mean spherical equivalent of postoperative refraction was −0.10 D (range −4.50 to +5.00 D). A clear visual axis was documented in the postoperative period by using imaging.

We conducted a retrospective, non-randomized study of 85 eyes from 56 patients who underwent cataract surgery with BIL IOL implantation via corneal incision (B. Lorenz et al., Giessen Pediatric Cataract Study Group, unpublished data). The patients were divided into four age groups, because we were convinced that there was a strong correlation between the preoperative age-specific condition of the eye and postoperative anatomical and functional results, which can influence the timing of the operation and application of the optimal surgical and therapeutic approach in the future. The distribution into age groups was as follows: 1st group, 0–younger than 3 months; 2nd group, 3 to 12 months; 3rd group, older than 12–36 months; and 4th group, older than 36 months to 17 years old. Unilateral cataracts were diagnosed in 24 cases (42.9%) and bilateral cataracts in 32 cases (57.1%). In three cases of bilateral cataract, only one eye was operated with the BIL technique.

The selected target refraction in cases of unilateral cataract was chosen by taking the refraction of the contralateral eye and the age at surgery into consideration. The highest dioptre power of the BIL IOL available in our operating facility was +34.5 D.

A clear visual axis was documented in all cases in the early postoperative period in our cohort (Fig. 22.1). The entire group's mean early postoperative refraction was +3.33 dioptres. However, it the different age groups and decreased gradually with age towards emmetropia from +9.76 D in the 1st age group to +0.39 D in 4th age group. The mean postoperative best corrected visual acuity (BCVA) in each group increased with age. The improvement of BCVA was significantly higher in older patients. Tromans et al. reported that the prediction error, meaning the difference between preoperative target refraction and postoperative achieved refraction, depended on axial length, corneal size and age at the time of surgery after lens-in-the-bag implantation [2]. Their results showed that the postoperative prediction error was larger in patients younger than 36 months of age and in patients with an AL of less than 20 mm.

We analysed the prediction error in four different age groups: according to age, axial length and corneal curvature. The prediction error in the different age groups decreased gradually from +3.43 D in the 1st group to +1.06 D in the 4th group (preliminary data) (Fig. 22.2). Our results correlate with previously reported data using the lens-in-the-bag technique and demonstrate an evident gradual decrease in prediction error with age at surgery. Similarly, we noticed a larger prediction error in eyes with shorter axial length and smaller corneal radius. This indicates that the standard formulas can be used with relative precision only in older paediatric patients, and new modified formulas have to be considered.

In our cohort, we analysed ten eyes of eight patients who had preoperative and postoperative astigmatism measurements to evaluate the significance of the main corneal incision's site 2.4 mm wide with respect to astigmatism changes. The mean preoperative astigmatism was −2.35 D (range −0.37 D to −8.00 D) with a mean axis of 36.5° (range 166° to 2°). Nine out of ten eyes had a temporal tunnel incision; one surgery was performed with a superior tunnel. The mean postoperative astigmatism was −1.55 D (range −0.5 D to −5.75 D) with a mean axis of 64.5° (range 180° to 4°). Nyström et al. reported the implantation of BIL IOL via a sclerocorneal incision. However, our data suggest that clear corneal or limbocorneal incision 2.4 mm wide does not induce a significant postoperative astigmatism once the resorbable sutures are gone.

The placement of both capsulorhexes into the optic groove facilitates the firm positioning of the BIL IOL with the possibility to implant toric IOLs in eyes with

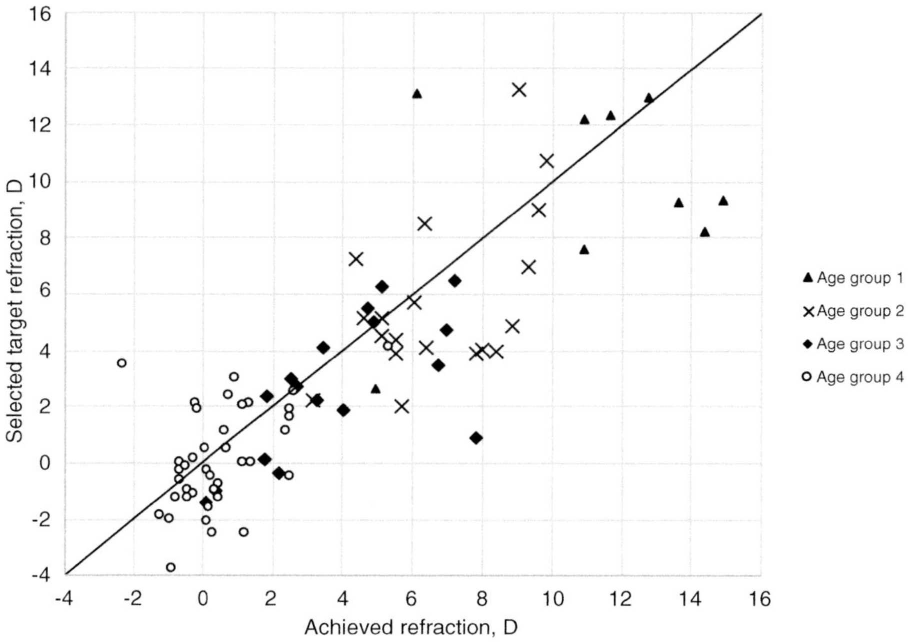

Fig. 22.2 Selected target refraction versus postoperative achieved refraction in different age groups (Giessen Pediatric Cataract Study Group, 85 eyes from 56 patients, unpublished data)

preexisting corneal astigmatism (see Chap. 11). However, there is a lack of data about the use of toric BIL IOL in children. In our study, we implanted the toric BIL IOL in both eyes of one patient. During the short-term follow-up (4 months), the position of the IOL remained stable, which was confirmed with autorefractometry.

22.1.3 Long-Term Visual Outcomes

In 2015, Van Looveren et al. reported the first long-term results of BIL IOL implantation during a 5-year follow-up period in 46 eyes of 31 children [13]. In their study, the authors enrolled patients aged 2 months to 14 years with various types of paediatric cataracts (including spherophakia and persistent foetal vasculature (PFV)). IOL calculations were based on the SRK/T formula using data from preoperative examinations performed under general anaesthesia. The target refraction in patients <3 months of age was +3.0 dioptres (D), 3–6 months, +2.0 D; and >6–9 months, +1.0 D. In patients older than 9 months, the target refraction was emmetropia. In cases with unilateral cataract, the target refraction was guided by the refraction of the contralateral eye. IOL power was available up to +39.0 D. The postoperative refraction ranged from −2.0 D to +2.0 D in 52% of cases. The refraction of the majority of cases tended to mild myopia with the highest result being −6.0 D. In 15 cases (30 eyes) of bilateral cataract, in which it was possible to determine preoperative visual acuity, the mean corrected distance visual acuity (CDVA) improved from 0.2 decimal preoperatively (range 0.0–0.4) to postoperative 0.83 decimal (range 0.2–1.0). In cases with unilateral cataract (16 children), the mean CDVA improved from 0.07 decimal (range 0.0 to 0.4) to postoperative 0.27 decimal (range 0.0–0.7) showing that maximum visual rehabilitation is more difficult to obtain in unilateral cases. The authors reported that the visual axis remained clear over the period of 5 years in 91.3% of the cases examined. Among the very few complications encountered, reopacifications occurred in four eyes of three children due to the inadequate placement of the posterior capsule into the IOL. These cases all required additional surgical intervention. Among the patients aged less than 6 months at the time of surgery (eight eyes of five patients), three eyes had no complication. The most common complications were reopacification of the visual axis and anterior synechia. The mean postoperative CDVA in patients younger than 6 months was 0.32 (decimal). The authors noted that reopacification, secondary glaucoma and inflammatory response were the main causes of a decrease of visual acuity in the long term. However, the rate of these complications was relatively low.

We analysed the long-term follow-up by the Giessen Pediatric Cataract Study Group (Lorenz et al., unpublished data). In our cohort of BIL IOL implantation, the longest follow-up period in the entire group of 56 patients (85 eyes) was 7 years. The mean postoperative follow-up was 16.2 months. A clear visual axis was documented in 94.1% of cases. In two cases (two eyes from the same patient), the visual axis was opaque due to postoperative uveal inflammation with opacification of the cornea and vitreous body. In the remaining cases, the cause of the opacification was retrolental proliferation as a result of inadequate position of the posterior capsulorhexis or insufficient separation of the posterior capsule from the anterior vitreous surface; this was treated surgically. The improvement of visual functions correlated with preoperative visual functions, ocular comorbidity, the compliance to amblyopia treatment and postoperative complications. In uncomplicated cases, a gradual increase in visual functions was noticed during the first 12 months after the surgery. Visual acuity continued to progress up until 72 months of follow-up.

Recently, Nyström et al. published their results in a series of 109 eyes of 84 children aged between 2 weeks and 14.1 years at the time of surgery. They found a clear visual axis in 95.4% of patients, over a mean follow-up of 2.8 years. Visual recovery was significantly better in children with bilateral cataracts as compared to unilateral cataracts. About 55.6% of eyes attained a CDVA of ≥0.5 decimal in the bilateral cataract group, as opposed to 37.5% in the unilateral cataract group [14].

As paediatric cataract is a relatively rare disease, paediatric patients are usually admitted to special eye departments where they undergo cataract surgery. Patients frequently travel hundreds of kilometres in order to obtain surgical care. After the treatment, a large contingent of the patients are followed up by local ophthalmologists in their native city or country, which makes it difficult to gather complete data on long-term results. The registration of the paediatric cases using a telemedicine approach should be considered.

22.2 Complications of the BIL IOL Technique

The visual outcomes following paediatric cataract surgery with the BIL technique are strongly related to surgical complications that can happen either during the surgery or in the postoperative period. Intra- and postoperative problems are typical to all kinds of cataract surgery with or without the implantation of intraocular lenses and in all age groups. It has been shown that the concept of BIL technique allows for the number of postoperative complications to decrease, such as PCO or macular oedema. Some of the complications occur because of intraoperative manipulations, while other complications are related to the anatomical and physiological characteristics of the developing paediatric eye. Among them are the small size of the anterior chamber, underdevelopment of the anterior chamber angle, short axial length, more active tissue response on surgical intervention and more.

In the following section, we describe paediatric cataract surgery's most important complications in general but more specifically with regard to the BIL technique.

22.2.1 Intraoperative Complications and Their Management

The operating field in neonates is characterized by a lack of space during any intraocular surgery. The reason for this is a small interpalpebral fissure and the relatively big ratio between the size of the cornea and sclera compared to the adult eye. We recommend a temporal approach in every case in order to reduce the difficulties encountered during surgery, thereby avoiding potential intrasurgical complications.

Congenital cataract can frequently be associated with microphthalmia and/or with eyelid malformation. If necessary, a canthotomy can be performed at the beginning of the surgery using Westcott scissors to make a single cut of 3–5 mm length.

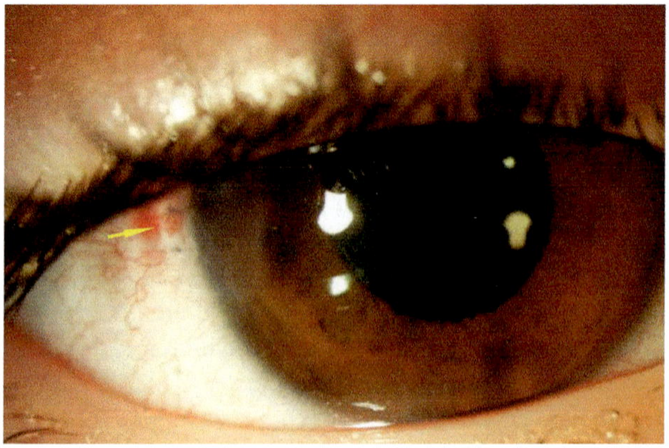

Fig. 22.3 Closure of the temporal limbo-corneal incision with 10.0 Vicryl suture (age at the time of surgery 7.6 years)

Even a small canthotomy will provide an adequate area in which to perform the intervention. The site of the cut does not usually bleed. At the end of the surgery, the canthotomy has to be closed using two to three absorbable single sutures. The site of canthotomy usually heals without any significant cosmetic defect.

Subconjunctival haemorrhages can occur during surgery. Bleeding from conjunctival or episcleral superficial vessels is usually limited due to the incomplete development of the vasculature in an infant's eye. The presence of this relatively minor complication can lead to major problems in the postoperative period. Perilimbal subconjunctival bleeding with elevation of the conjunctiva can impact the closure of the entry wound, even if it has been sutured. Continuous bleeding can cause the leakage of the blood into the anterior chamber when the wound margins are not very tight. Suturing of the operating wounds is strongly advocated as cataract incisions in children are rarely self-sealing (Fig. 22.3). Additionally, a subconjunctival haemorrhage can serve as a medium for bacterial growth. Massive and continuous conjunctival bleeding should be stopped using diathermy. A subconjunctival haemorrhage can be an issue by which the parents of the patient judge the surgery's success. This is why it is important in such cases to show the unpatched eye after the surgery to the parents and explain the natural course of the healing process.

Surgical Trauma of the Cornea Like in every cataract surgery, complications related to wound construction can occur when performing the BIL technique (Fig. 22.4). It should be borne in mind that the incisions will not self-seal at the end of the surgery in a child's eye, even if hydrated, due to the thin cornea, low rigidity of cornea and sclera and the softness of the eye. The clear corneal, limbocorneal or sclerocorneal incisions have to be performed in a three-step manner. We perform an initial limbocorneal incision 2.2 mm wide, and we extend it to 2.4 mm just before the implantation of the BIL IOL. If the incision tears, it will influence the surgery flow, and the incision has to be sutured immediately, and a new incision should be made elsewhere if necessary. We use 23- and 25-gauge MVR blades to create the

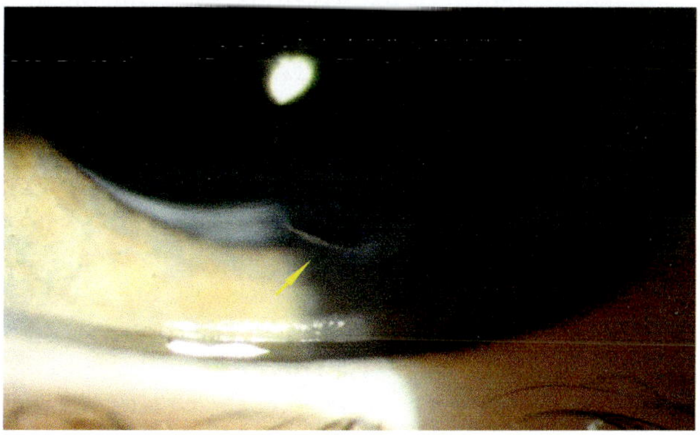

Fig. 22.4 Corneal damage after pediatric cataract surgery (age at the time of surgery 6 months)

paracenteses, as this is sufficient for the use of micro-instruments, and the risks of postoperative wound leak are, therefore, reduced.

Improper wound construction can facilitate iris prolapse and result in postoperative pupillary defects, as well as uveal reaction. Therefore, the length of the incisions ought to be long enough to prevent prolapse of the iris. Iris prolapse has to be treated with iris reposition, and an alternative wound creation should be considered. All incisions should be sutured and tested for leakage at the end of surgery (Fig. 22.3).

Small Pupil and Iris Maldevelopment Adequate mydriasis is essential for any cataract surgery, especially during the implantation of a BIL IOL. The diameter of the optical part of the BIL IOL (type 89A) is 5 mm, and the total diameter is 7.5 mm. The minimal pupil size has to be 5.5–6.5 mm in diameter in order to visualize the capsulorhexes and the edges of the IOL during implantation. To achieve sufficient mydriasis, additional intracameral injection of diluted mydriatics (adrenalin) can be necessary. However, this step has to be discussed with the anaesthesiologist due to possible cardiovascular reaction even on a low concentration of mydriatics.

Different iris retracting devices can also be used in order to reach a stable size of the pupil during the whole surgery. Temporary implantation of iris retractors can be considered, which will necessitate four to six additional paracenteses. An MVR blade is preferred over a 27-gauge needle for this purpose, because a needle creates a round-shaped incision with poorer adaptation of the opening, as opposed to the slit incision of a blade. The iris retractors can damage the pigment of the pupillary margin, due to the small contact surface and relatively strong retraction. This can lead to an irregular pupil after the surgery and to the dispersion of pigmented cells within the anterior chamber and onto the IOL surface.

Alternatively, iris retracting devices such as the Visitec® I-Ring® Pupil Expander (Beaver-Visitec International, Inc., Waltham, MA, USA), the Malyugin Ring 2.0 (MicroSurgical Technology, Redmond, WA, USA) or similar iris expanders can be used. However, the use of iris expanders is limited in younger children because of the small size of their eyes. We recommend using the iris expanders only in eyes with a corneal diameter of over 10 mm.

Maldevelopment of the iris is not a contraindication for BIL IOL implantation. In case of iris coloboma or aniridia, the visualization of the capsular bag and retrolental space is improved (Fig. 22.5). It can help during the implantation of the BIL IOL and avoid possible side effects of intracameral miotics. Nonetheless, partial or complete absence of the iris can influence the postoperative visual function and cause increased light sensitivity.

Capsulorhexis-Related Complications The creation of an anterior and posterior continuous curvilinear capsulorhexis (ACCC and PCCC) is essential for the successful implantation of a BIL IOL. The capsular anatomy is different in paediatric patients than it is in adults. The vastly increased elasticity of the capsular bag, a more anterior insertion of the zonulae and a higher vitreous pressure make both the

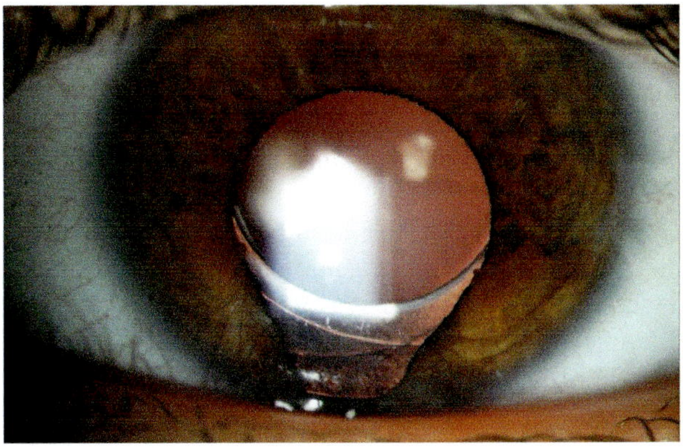

Fig. 22.5 BIL IOL implanted in the eye with coloboma of the iris (age at the time of surgery 12 months)

anterior and the posterior capsulorhexes less predictable and reproducible in children [13, 14]. These circumstances increase the risk of capsulorhexis-related complications. Understanding of the capsules' behaviour can be gained through building up own experience.

Radial tearing of the anterior capsulorhexis may not only complicate a planned BIL IOL implantation but can also lead to more severe complications, such as rupture of the posterior capsule and vitreous prolapse. In case of an extended anterior capsular tear, the use of a BIL IOL has to be reconsidered. However, the BIL IOL can be gently implanted when only a limited tear of the anterior or posterior capsulorhexis has occurred. The implantation of a BIL IOL Type 89F with larger optic and extended anterior haptic element that can cover a capsular defect should be considered in the case of limited capsular rupture in older paediatric patients.

Adequately filling the anterior chamber with ophthalmic viscoelastic device (OVD) is recommended in order to avoid the tearing of the anterior capsulorhexis. The flap of the capsulorhexis has to be inverted backwards and pulled towards the centre of the pupil or directed even a little bit in the opposite direction of the rhexis. In case of the extension of the capsulorhexis, anterior chamber scissors or vitreoretinal small gauge scissors can be used to direct and correct the extension of the capsulorhexis.

The size of the capsulorhexis has to be somewhat smaller to the targeted size. In our experience, the anterior capsulorhexis is more predictable with the smaller caliper ring #4 (4.3 mm), while the rhexis is still big enough to implant the BIL IOL without overstretching both the anterior and posterior capsulorhexes.

Zonular dehiscence can be a sign of the maldevelopment of the zonular apparatus or ocular trauma and can sometimes be diagnosed only during surgery. A capsular tension ring can be used in cases of limited zonular dialysis. Tassignon et al. reported the use of bean-shaped rings (Morcher GmbH, Stuttgart, Germany), the additional supporting elements produced by PMMA, that can stabilize and centre the BIL IOL [15]. These can also be considered in case of sectorial zonular dehiscence.

Incomplete Separation of the Anterior Vitreous and Vitreous Prolapse The separation of the anterior hyaloid from the posterior capsule is an important step in the surgery. As initially described by Tassignon et al., the main goal of injecting hyaluronic acid through the incision in the posterior capsule is to push the anterior hyaloid posteriorly and displace the posterior capsule forwards so that it will reach the anterior capsulorhexis [10]. Another important issue of this manoeuvre is to make the posterior capsule, as well as the edge of the future posterior capsulorhexis, free of vitreous adhesions in order to perform the placement of both capsulorhexes into the BIL IOL groove without difficulties. To avoid complications, the injection of the OVD between the posterior capsule and the anterior vitreous should be done gently while directing the injection flow towards the periphery of the capsular bag, but not into the vitreous cavity. In children with cataract, there is an increased incidence of anomalous anatomy of the vitreo-lenticular interface. This can make the separation of anterior hyaloid from the posterior capsule more difficult. In cases where it is impossible to perform an adequate separation, a partial vitrectomy may help to free the posterior capsulorhexis from strongly adhesive vitreous.

An incomplete separation of the anterior vitreous from the posterior capsule can cause a vitreous prolapse. In this case, the prolapsed vitreous has to be removed from the anterior and posterior chamber with an anterior vitrectomy before positioning the BIL implant. An injection of a small amount of triamcinolone acetonide can help to detect the prolapsed vitreous. We experienced a vitreous prolapse in 14.1% of cases of our paediatric patients (12 eyes). The most frequent causes of vitreous prolapse were the presence of remaining fetal vasculature and fibrosis of the posterior capsule and posterior capsular tear. In all 12 cases, a limited anterior vitrectomy was performed and the BIL IOL was successfully implanted.

22.2.2 Postoperative Complications and Their Management

Corneal oedema appears to be one of the most common complications but is usually transient. The surgery itself, as it is performed within the very small space of the anterior and posterior chamber of the child's eye, is the most frequent cause of corneal oedema. Additionally, postoperative inflammation, as well as ocular hypertension, can lead to dysfunction of the endothelial cells and swelling of the stroma. An incidence rate of 35% temporary corneal oedema has been reported in paediatric cataract surgery. However, as a rule, it resolves spontaneously within 3–5 days without treatment.

Deformation of the Pupil and Capture of the Iris Postoperative inflammatory reaction as well as intrasurgical trauma to the iris can lead to formation of anterior synechia and deformation of the pupil (Fig. 22.6). Surgical reconstruction of the pupil has to be considered in the early postoperative period in order to prevent iris atrophy, corneal opacification and increased light sensitivity.

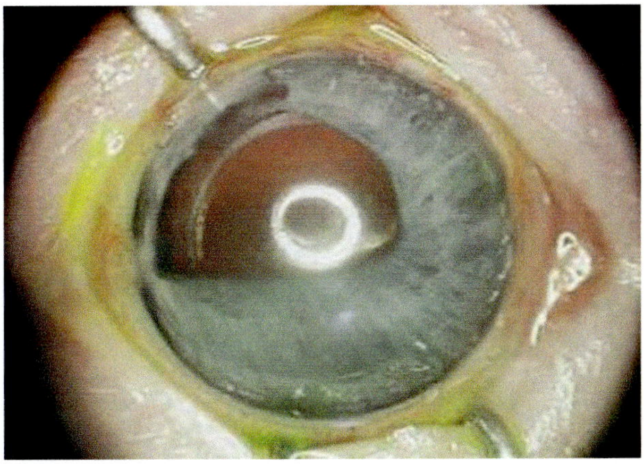

Fig. 22.6 Deformation of the iris after BIL IOL implantation with anterior synechia connected to the sites of paracentesis (age at the time of surgery 3.8 months)

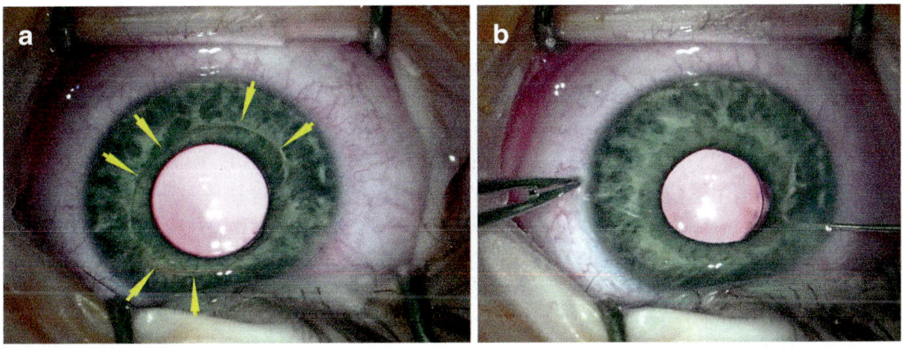

Fig. 22.7 Circular iriscapture in early postoperative period after implantation BIL IOL Type 89A (**a**). Surgical reposition of the iris in the same patient (**b**) (age at the time of surgery 2.7 years)

Spontaneous constriction of a previously dilated pupil can lead to iris capture into the groove of BIL IOL in the postoperative period (Fig. 22.7). In our patients, we noticed that an injection of air into the anterior chamber at the end of the surgery can lead to iris capture as well. To prevent an iris capture, intraoperative pupillary constriction using a miotic agent for intraocular use (such as acetylcholine or carbachol) is recommended after correct placement of the BIL IOL. In the early postoperative period, instillation of pilocarpine 1% should be considered in patients with exceptionally large pupils.

Longstanding and untreated capture of the iris can result in synechiae which can lead to degenerative and ischemic changes of the pupillary rim. This will result in an irregular pupil with reduced constriction ability. Freshly diagnosed cases of iris capture can sometimes be treated with topical mydriatics, enabling the iris to escape from the groove of the implant. An additional surgical intervention is preferable when synechiae are already present. This will then consist of the injection of OVD, release of iris capture and injection of a miotic agent in the anterior chamber.

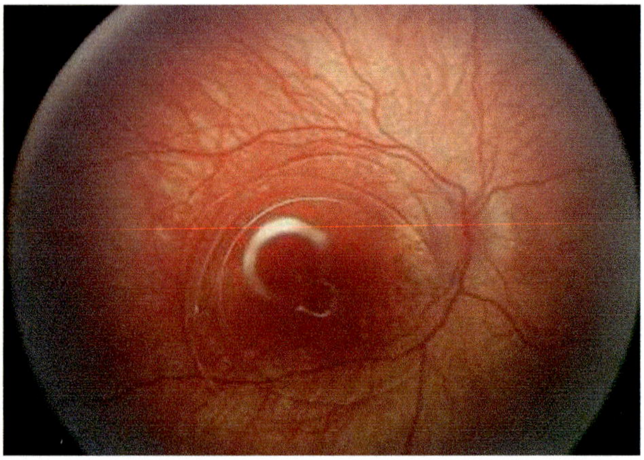

Fig. 22.8 Dislocation of BIL IOL into the vitreous cavity due to inadequate size of capsulorhexis (age at the time of surgery 3.8 months)

Dislocation of the BIL IOL The main causes of IOL dislocation are an incorrect placement of the capsular bag into the groove of the IOL, an oversized capsulorhexis (>5.3 mm), shallow anterior chamber after the surgery and ocular trauma.

In our series of cases, we documented only one case of IOL dislocation into the vitreous cavity, in spite of the calliper ring being used to facilitate the anterior capsulorhexis (Fig. 22.8). In this case, after vitreous removal, the IOL was explanted through the corneal incision, and a three-piece posterior chamber IOL was implanted into the sulcus with capsular support. We did not record any cases of dislocation of the BIL IOL into the anterior chamber.

Decentration of the BIL IOL Optimal centration of the central optical zone of the BIL IOL is necessary to achieve the best corrected visual acuity after surgery. The centration of the BIL IOL depends on the centration of anterior and posterior capsulorhexes. IOL decentration is, therefore, related primarily to complications concerning the capsulorhexis. Furthermore, fibrosis of the capsular bag with retrolental vitreous proliferation and improper separation of the anterior vitreous from the posterior capsule may play a role in complicated cases.

The careful positioning and creation of both anterior and posterior capsulorhexes are essential to obtaining a good position for the IOL (see Chaps. 7 and 8). Verbruggen et al. have studied BIL IOL centration in adult patients. The decentration of BIL IOL was less when compared to other study results that evaluated lens-in-the-bag IOLs [16]. The authors concluded that the fibrotic changes of the capsular bag have no significant effect on BIL IOL centration in the postoperative period.

Ocular Hypotony According to the American Academy of Ophthalmology (AAO), a decrease of intraocular pressure below the normal limit (<10 mm Hg) is classified as postoperative ocular hypotony (in adults).

The most common cause of postoperative hypotony is the leakage of aqueous humour through one or more incisions. Additionally, hypotony can appear as a result of postoperative uveitis, cyclodialysis or retinal detachment. The flattening of the anterior chamber is the most frequent sign of postoperative hypotony.

Biomicroscopy with a cobalt filter and the instillation of 1–2 drops of 2% fluorescein (Seidel test) are usually performed in order to detect the site of the leakage. Careful examination of the wounds has to be performed 24–48 h after the primary surgery. Additional closure using 10.0 Vicryl or Prolene is recommended in case of postoperative leakage through a wound. Ultrasound examination has to be performed in order to exclude cyclodialysis or retinal detachment. Chronic uveitis can also cause ocular hypotony in the late postoperative period.

Ocular Hypertension Glaucoma-related adverse events are common in paediatric cataract surgery. The risk of glaucoma persists in spite of the improvement in surgical techniques, but the implantation of an IOL does not increase the rate of postoperative ocular hypertension. It has been reported that glaucoma-related complications appear more frequently in younger patients within the first year of follow-up, especially when the surgery is performed during the first weeks of life. Ocular hypertension is also more likely to develop in patients with bilateral cataracts. A longer follow-up of these children may further characterize risk factors and long-term outcomes.

The implantation of the BIL IOL creates no additional risks of postoperative ocular hypertension in paediatric patients. However, the haptic of the BIL IOL in eyes with microphthalmia may lead to contact with underdeveloped structures of the anterior chamber angle. Tassignon et al. reported two cases of ocular hypertension in their case series [12]. Both cases were reported to suffer from additional anterior segment dysgenesis. Medical treatment was applied in one case, while a surgical procedure was needed in the other. In the same centre, Van Looveren et al. reported one case of glaucoma in their series with a 5-year follow-up [13]. Nyström et al. reported glaucoma in 13.8% percent of eyes, in line with other recent reports in paediatric cataract surgery [14]. In this study, a postoperative IOP higher than 22 mmHg was considered as glaucoma.

We analysed the postoperative glaucoma-associated adverse events in different age groups (Giessen Pediatric Cataract Study Group). An intraocular eye pressure above 18 mmHg, measured with applanation tonometry, was considered to be ocular hypertension. The highest rate of increased IOP (33.3%) was seen in the youngest group of patients where the surgery was performed before 3 months of age. The rates of ocular hypertension in older groups were as follows: 6.3% between 3 and 12 months, 23.5% above 12 months to 36 months, and 16.1% over 36 months. In the entire group (85 eyes of 56 patients), the rate of ocular hypertension after the surgery was 18.8% (16 eyes) (B. Lorenz et al., unpublished data). A topical medications or surgical intervention were needed to control IOP in 16.5% of cases in entire group (14 eyes).

As a first-choice medication, carbonic anhydrase inhibitors or topical betablockers are advocated. When medical treatment is insufficient, surgical treatment can become necessary. Glaucoma-related adverse events can occur years after the cataract surgery; therefore, strict follow-up with regular IOP measurements is highly recommended.

The method to measure IOP in children has to be considered as well as age-related features of the ocular tissues. We recommend using Goldmann or Perkins applanation tonometry and comparing the values with those from an iCare tonometer. In many cases of paediatric cataract, an efficient applanation tonometry is only possible under general anaesthesia. Lowering of the IOP, due to medications used for general anaesthesia, has to be taken into account while assessing the IOP values.

Postoperative glaucoma-associated adverse events should be expected in eyes with abnormalities of the anterior chamber angle prior to surgery. While the patients are in narcosis, we perform a contact gonioscopy using a RetCam II (Clarity Medical Systems, Pleasanton, CA, USA) in each case. Discovering an abnormal development of the anterior chamber angle preoperatively can forecast the postoperative IOL fluctuation and can influence the surgical approach, as well as the postoperative follow-up regime.

Reopacification of the Visual Axis After BIL IOL Implantation The main advantage of the BIL technique is that the anterior and posterior capsules are placed into the groove of the BIL IOL. This keeps any residual lens epithelial cells in a closed space, which also decreases the risk of retrolental reopacification of the visual axis considerably. Tassignon et al. have described rare cases of retrolental reopacification caused by the improper placement of the posterior capsulorhexis. They stated that in spite of the presence of the posterior capsulorhexis, the lens epithelial cells can proliferate onto the surface of the anterior vitreous from the free and uncaptured remnants of the posterior capsule. In these cases, the posterior capsulorhexis was easily placed back into the groove of the BIL IOL after the removal of the opacities with vitrectomy.

In our cohort, we diagnosed retrolental reopacification in few cases in long-term follow-up, which was treated with BIL IOL reposition and vitrectomy. Moreover, in our series we observed two cases with the presence of pigmented precipitates on the anterior surface of the BIL IOL in the late postoperative period. A possible explanation could be the release of the pigmented cells from the iris during or after surgery, especially in small eyes. However, whether these small precipitates have a negative influence on the visual functions remains questionable.

The appearance of deposits or precipitates of calcium and phosphate in the BIL IOL biomaterial has been described previously. However, it is possible to explant a damaged BIL IOL and to implant a new one [17]. The correct placement of the BIL IOL can be re-examined postoperatively by using hand-held or standard optic coherence tomography systems.

Postoperative Uveitis and Endophthalmitis Surgical trauma and an immature blood-ocular barrier predispose children to excessive, non-specific uveal reactions in the postoperative period. The grade of inflammation can vary from singular cells seen in the anterior chamber to excessive fibrin reactions with the formation of anterior and posterior synechia, secondary glaucoma and vitreal exudation. Perioperative trauma of the iris and ciliary body can play a crucial role in the development of postoperative uveitis.

Postoperative inflammation can be prevented and treated with steroids, NSAID and irrigation of the anterior chamber with heparin and by minimizing surgical trauma.

In BIL surgery, the amount of residual lens epithelial cells that can be released and float in the anterior chamber is reduced compared to the lens-in-the-bag technique. This might decrease the risk of postoperative uveitis in compromised cases.

In our study, we observed excessive postoperative granulomatous uveitis with membrane formation in two eyes from the same patient. Surgical removal of the fibrin membranes was needed in one eye, while the other eye was treated conservatively first and was then operated on for secondary glaucoma.

A postoperative infectious endophthalmitis may occur as a devastating complication in rare cases of paediatric cataract. This has an incidence rate of 0.071–0.45%. The presence of ocular or systemic infection, as well as intraoperative complications such as improper wound construction, iris prolapse and vitreous loss with prolonged surgery time, is a risk factor in the development of endophthalmitis. Nasolacrimal duct obstruction and upper respiratory tract infection have to be excluded before surgery as they can create an additional risk for postoperative endophthalmitis. The prophylaxis and treatment approaches of acute postoperative endophthalmitis in children are similar to those in adults. The use of intracameral antibiotics at the end of the surgery is strongly recommended. The incidence of endophthalmitis in paediatric BIL surgery has not been reported on. However, the possible risk factors must be considered nonetheless.

Cystoid macular oedema (CME) is considered to be caused by intraoperative and/or postoperative release of cytokines and vitreoretinal traction. This can lead to the disruption of the inner blood-retinal barrier resulting in the accumulation of intraretinal fluid within the inner retinal layers. Other pathophysiologic mechanisms include intraocular inflammation, phototoxic trauma and postoperative ocular hypotony. Optical coherence tomography is considered to be the gold standard in establishing the diagnosis of CME. The diagnosis of CME in paediatric patients using OCT can be challenging due to compliance issues and can result in underdiagnosis. We use a hand-held OCT (Bioptigen, Morrisville, NC, USA) after the surgery and during the follow-up to eventually detect macular oedema in our paediatric patients. The advantage of this approach is that an experienced examiner can perform OCT scanning without general anaesthesia. We have not observed CME in any of our cases. In some patients, absence of the normal foveal indentation can be revealed as an additional finding, indicating a more complex ocular pathology, which might have a possible impact on the final visual outcome.

The incidence of CME in paediatric patients is reported to be low, possibly due to the anatomical particularities of a child's eye, such as a tight vitreoretinal adhesion, but maybe also underdiagnosed. During the BIL technique, the anterior vitreous is separated from the posterior capsule using viscodissection. This minimizes the anterior displacement of the vitreous and might lower the risk of CME. There are no cases of CME reported in paediatric patients who underwent BIL surgery.

Vitreous haemorrhage (VH) occurs rarely in paediatric cataract surgery and can be caused by accidental ocular hypotony or iatrogenic trauma to vascularized tissues. The source of the haemorrhage can include the fetal vasculature of the iris, ciliary body or anterior chamber angle. Occasionally, when an excessive conjunctival haemorrhage is present, the blood can leak through the corneal incisions into the anterior chamber and vitreous cavity. The main predisposing factor for vitreous haemorrhage is the presence of persistent fetal vasculature (PFV). A mild VH usually resolves spontaneously over 2–4 weeks. In the case of dense VH, a surgical removal of the vitreous with the PPV approach has to be considered. In our group of patients, we did not see any case of VH after BIL IOL implantation.

Retinal detachment (RD) remains one of the most dangerous complications that can appear following cataract surgery in children and has an incidence of about 1%. The pathogenesis of RD is not entirely clear. The presence of pathologic myopia, peripheral retinal degeneration, displacement of the lens or a history of ocular trauma can increase the risk of RD in children. Intraoperative complications, such as capsular bag loss, luxation of the lens into the vitreous cavity, vitreous haemorrhage and vitreous prolapse, can also lead to RD. There were no incidences of retinal detachment in a long-term follow-up study of BIL IOL implantation in children [13]. We also have not observed any case of RD in our group of paediatric cataracts operated with BIL IOL (B. Lorenz et al., unpublished data). The management of RD in children includes the standard surgical approaches, such as PPV and scleral buckling. Proliferative vitreoretinopathy (PVR) and detachment of the macula can lead to a poor prognosis of visual recovery.

Choroidal detachment is a rare complication as well. The fluctuation of IOP during surgery and in the postoperative period can result in dilatation of choroidal vessels with effusion of plasma into the subchoroidal space. Choroidal detachment alone or in association with subchoroidal haemorrhage has not yet been reported in paediatric BIL patients.

22.3 Core Messages

- Careful follow-up and monitoring of visual function and amblyopia is essential to obtaining good outcomes in the long term.
- The bag-in-the-lens technique allows for the minimization of the rate of visual axis reopacification after cataract surgery in children.
- The BIL technique does not otherwise present considerable differences in intra- or postoperative complication rates compared to conventional surgery techniques.

References

1. Kuhli-Hattenbach C, Hofmann C, Wenner Y, Koch F, Kohnen T. Congenital cataract surgery without intraocular lens implantation in persistent fetal vasculature syndrome: long-term clinical and functional results. J Cataract Refract Surg. 2016;42:759–67.
2. Tromans C, Haigh PM, Biswas S, Lloyd IC. Accuracy of intraocular lens power calculation in paediatric cataract surgery. Br J Ophthalmol. 2001;85:939–41.
3. Andreo LK, Wilson ME, Saunders RA. Predictive value of regression and theoretical IOL formulas in paediatric intraocular lens implantation. J Pediatr Ophthalmol Strabismus. 1997;34(4):240–3.
4. Lambert SR, Lyons CJ, editors. Taylor and Hoyt's pediatric ophthalmology and strabismus. 5th ed. Amsterdam, The Netherlands: Elsevier; 2017.
5. Lin AA, Buckley EG. Update on pediatric cataract surgery and intraocular lens implantation. Curr Opin Ophthalmol. 2010;21:55–9.
6. Trivedi RH, Wilson ME, Vasavada AR, Shah SK, Vasaveda V, Vasaveda VA. Visual axis opacification after cataract surgery and hydrophobic acrylic intraocular lens implantation in the first year of life. J Cataract Refract Surg. 2011;37:83–7.
7. Tassignon MJ, De Groot V, Smets RME, Tawab B, Vervecken F. Secondary closure of posterior continuous curvilinear capsulorhexis. J Cataract Refract Surg. 1996;22:1200–5.
8. Tassignon MJ, De Groot V, Vervecken F, van Tenten Y. Secondary closure of posterior continuous curvilinear capsulorhexis in normal eyes and eyes at risk for postoperative inflammation. J Cataract Refract Surg. 1998;24:1333–133.
9. Vasavada AR, Praveen MR, Tassignon M-J, Shah SK, Vasavada VA, Vasavada VA, Van Looveren J, De Veuster I, Trivedi RH. Posterior capsule management in congenital cataract surgery. J Cataract Refract Surg. 2011;37:173–93.
10. Tassignon MJ, De Groot V, Vrensen GF. Bag-in-the-lens implantation of intraocular lenses. J Cataract Refract Surg. 2002;28:1182–8.
11. Werner L, Tassignon MJ, Gobin L, Rozema J, Davis D, Brubaker J. Bag-in-the-lens: first pathological analysis of a human eye obtained postmortem. J Cataract Refract Surg. 2008;34:2163–5.
12. Tassignon M-J, De Veuster I, Godts D, Kosec D, Van den Dooren K, Gobin L. Bag-in-the-lens intraocular lens implantation in the pediatric eye. J Cataract Refract Surg. 2007;33:611–7.
13. Van Looveren J, et al. Pediatric bag-in-the-lens intraocular lens implantation: long-term follow-up. J Cataract Refract Surg. 2015;41:1685–92.
14. Nyström A, Almarzouki N, Magnusson G, Zetterberg M. Phacoemulsification and primary implantation with bag-in-the-lens intraocular lens in children with unilateral and bilateral cataract. Acta Ophthalmol. 2018.; jan 19 (epub;96:364.
15. Tassignon M-J, Dhubhghaill SN. Bean-shaped ring segments for capsule stretching and centration of bag-in-the-lens cataract surgery. J Cataract Refract Surg. 2014;40:8–12.
16. Verbruggen KHM. Intraocular lens centration and visual outcomes after bag-in-the-lens implantation. J Cataract Refract Surg. 2007;33:1267–72.
17. Ní Dhubhghaill S, Van Os L, De Keizer RJ, Taal M, Zakaria N, Tassignon MJ. Intraocular lens exchange technique for an opacified bag-in-the-lens. J Cataract Refract Surg. 2015;41:924–8.

Printed by Printforce, the Netherlands